THE LITTLE BOOK OF

Sleep
Meditations

THE LITTLE BOOK OF SLEEP MEDITATIONS

An Hachette UK Company
www.hachette.co.uk

Vie Books, an imprint of Summersdale Publishers
Part of Octopus Publishing Group Limited
Carmelite House
50 Victoria Embankment
LONDON
EC4Y 0DZ
UK

www.summersdale.com

The authorized representative in the EEA is Hachette Ireland, 8 Castlecourt Centre, Dublin 15, D15 XTP3, Ireland (email: info@hbgi.ie)

Printed and bound in China

ISBN: 978-1-83799-558-5
eISBN: 978-1-83799-559-2

This FSC® label means that materials and other controlled sources used for the product have been responsibly sourced

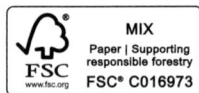

FSC
www.fsc.org

MIX
Paper | Supporting
responsible forestry
FSC® C016973

Substantial discounts on bulk quantities of Summersdale books are available to corporations, professional associations and other organizations. For details contact general enquiries: telephone: +44 (0) 1243 771107 or email: enquiries@summersdale.com.

THE LITTLE BOOK OF

Sleep
Meditations

*Mindfulness Exercises
to Help You Sleep*

ANNIE FAY MEITCHIK

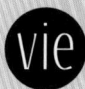

vie

CONTENTS

Introduction

Whether you're regularly struggling to sleep or want to fully benefit from those precious moments of rest, you will find dozens of mindful meditations and useful tips throughout this book. Consider these pages as a safe space for you to return to whenever you're looking to unwind, reset and focus on self-care.

Numerous studies have shown how important sleep is for our mental, emotional and physical well-being; however, many of us still struggle to wake up feeling energized – the 2019 Philips Global Sleep Survey showed that 62 per cent of adults around the world are not sleeping as well as they would like to.

Thankfully, if you're part of this majority, the exercises in these pages can help alleviate common sleep problems and enhance your well-being by providing you with new ways to approach your bedtime routine. By learning how meditation and other mindfulness rituals can help you to relax, you may even find that this book will start to positively affect your days as well as

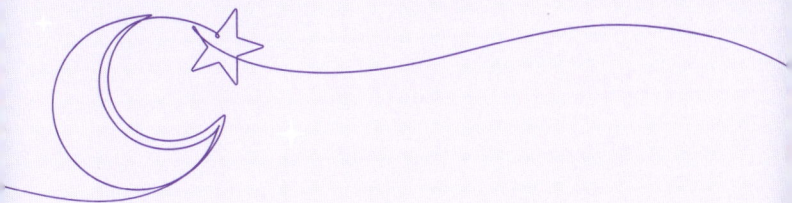

your nights. When we are well rested, we are better equipped to enter the world with joy, inner peace and a stronger sense of presence.

So, welcome to *The Little Book of Sleep Meditations*, where you'll begin your journey toward a calmer, more restful night's sleep.

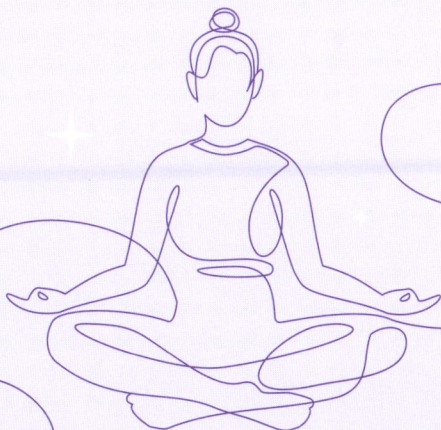

CHAPTER ONE:

Before
We Begin

LAYING THE FOUNDATION

Sleep is essential to maintain good mental, emotional and physical well-being. Yet, how can we go about mastering the art of sleeping to get the most out of our rest?

This book offers a variety of tips, suggestions for evening rituals, and information regarding the science of sleep. Understanding why we rest, how our sleep cycles work, and what causes us to struggle to fall or stay asleep will help us become better informed about our own bedtime routines.

The meditation exercises presented can be completed in 5, 10 or 15 minutes by following step-by-step directions, allowing you to experiment and then choose what works best for you. While some meditations are best practised before bed when you're ready to fall asleep, others can help you fall back to sleep, and many can be adapted to practise during the day in any environment where you can safely and comfortably pause for a few minutes. Some of the exercises are geared toward falling asleep in general, while others will help you focus on and let go of particular things that may be causing you stress.

What causes disturbed sleep and inability to fall asleep?

Before we begin, it's important to understand what causes issues with sleep. If you're struggling to fall asleep or stay asleep, or finding yourself feeling tired every day, please know you are not alone. While it can be worthwhile to consult with a healthcare professional, many issues related to sleep also have to do with stress. Yet, our busy lifestyles can make it hard for us to slow down and reflect on how things like our work or relationships are affecting us. Below are a few common causes of sleep struggles:

- Drinking caffeinated beverages or alcohol too close to bedtime
- Eating or snacking shortly before trying to fall asleep
- Inconsistency in your schedule or an inability to go to sleep and wake up around the same times each day
- Mental and physical health issues
- Screen time in bed
- Stress (financial, work, family, relationships, studying, etc.)

While some of these common causes are easier to address, like not drinking coffee before bed, things like stress can be harder to manage. Meditation and self-care rituals can be great ways to alleviate roadblocks to restfulness, but chronic stress should be treated with the advice of a therapist or other forms of professional help.

What are sleep cycles?

When learning more about sleep, it is important to understand the interplay between how many hours of sleep you need and sleep cycles. Even if you are sleeping for eight or more hours a night, for rest to feel truly beneficial, the body needs to go through four different sleep stages. These stages allow you to fully gain the restorative benefits of sleep.

1. Stage One, often referred to as N1, occurs when you first fall asleep. Body and brain activities are just beginning to slow down, making this the transition between being awake and drifting off.

2. Stage Two, often referred to as N2, is when you start to fall into a deeper sleep and brain activity continues to slow down.

3. Stage Three, or N3, is known as "deep sleep", when your brain activity goes into a pattern of delta waves (see p.142). This stage is key to having restorative sleep that can help boost immunity and even help with creativity and memory.

4. Stage Four is what many of us are most familiar with: REM (rapid eye movement) sleep. REM sleep is associated with dreaming and is when brain activity increases. Once these four stages are complete, the cycle starts over and repeats usually around four to six times.

These four distinct sleep stages ensure your brain and body are getting the rest they need to develop and reset each day.

Creating a calm sleeping environment

When you're struggling to sleep, you want your bedroom to feel as inviting and comfortable as possible. Often, our bedrooms can unintentionally become dumping grounds for laundry that needs folding, clutter we don't want to leave in communal spaces, and other distractions. Fortunately, there are many things you can do to create a sleeping environment that feels welcoming and calm. These things can help signal to your brain that entering your bedroom means you are ready to unwind and sleep.

Some ways in which you can create a calm sleeping environment include:

- **A tidy bedroom:** Always make your bed in the morning so it is inviting to get into in the evening. Ensure that the space is clean and clear of distractions.

- **Alarm clock:** Using an old-school alarm clock can be a great way to help you to wake up at a desired time if you want your bedroom to be a no-phone zone.

- **Aromatherapy:** Smell is an extremely powerful sense. By burning incense or using an oil diffuser before bed you can train your brain to associate the smell of lavender, for example, with sleep.

- **Bedding:** Invest in bedding that is cosy for you and allows you to sleep at a temperature most conducive to your restfulness.

- **Blackout blinds or curtains:** Sunlight or city lights streaming in through your windows can wake you or keep you up when you're trying to sleep. Blackout blinds or curtains can effectively darken your space.

Avoiding bright lights and electronics

Melatonin is a hormone that helps with sleep and balancing our circadian rhythms (the body and brain's internal clock over a period of 24 hours). The brain produces melatonin in response to darkness, which is why screen time is not ideal around bedtime. The blue light from our phones, tablets, computers or televisions can actually block melatonin production, throwing off our circadian rhythms.

Technology has vastly changed the way we live. We can often find ourselves plugged into our phones and computers, checking through our emails and striving to accomplish as much as we can during the day... and even into the evening. Bringing these devices and activities into the bedroom can contribute to difficulty sleeping.

If you're struggling with sleep, consider whether you often use devices with blue light in bed and try some of these easy adjustments:

1. **Airplane mode or "Do not disturb":** Use these features so your phone doesn't buzz or light up with notifications through the night.

2. **Night mode:** Most electronics have settings which enable you to adjust to a night mode, changing the blue light to a warmer light. Try setting this to automatically turn on in the evenings and reset in the mornings, or simply keep your devices on a warmer setting all the time to reduce the strain on your eyes.

3. **Time limits:** Set time limits so that your device automatically turns off at a certain time – which is useful if watching things helps you fall asleep.

ALTERNATIVES TO SCREENS BEFORE BED

While there are ways to reduce the effect screens can have on us before bed, there are also plenty of other activities you can explore if you'd like to avoid using electronics to fall asleep.

Studies have shown that reading a book before bed can help de-stimulate the brain, alleviate stress and enhance sleep quality. While a book may seem like the most obvious alternative to a screen, there are many offline activities you can experiment with to discover what works best for you.

- Colouring or drawing
- Completing activities in a puzzle book
- Crocheting or knitting
- Journalling
- Following a guided meditation
- Listening to a podcast
- Listening to an audiobook
- Listening to soft music

Perfecting your bedside table

After a long day, it feels wonderful to get into bed knowing that anything you might need during the night is to hand. How many times have you started to drift off, only to realize your throat is a little dry, or you forgot to plug your phone in to charge?

If you often find yourself getting into bed only to remember you have left something you needed in another room or out of reach, try to get into the habit of placing any items you might need on your bedside table beforehand.

Here are some possible essentials to get you started:

- Book
- Chargers
- Notebook and pen
- Pillow spray
- Sleep mask
- Water

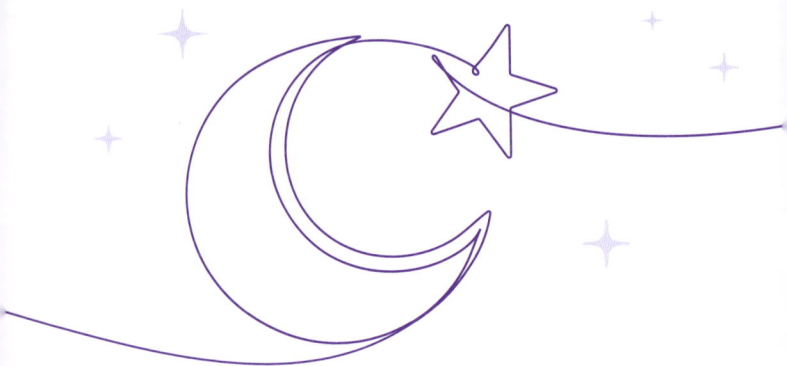

*Sleep is the golden
chain that ties health and
our bodies together.*

THOMAS DEKKER

COLD EXPOSURE

You may be familiar with some of the benefits of ice plunges, but did you know cold-water exposure can be beneficial to sleep?

The shock you experience from cold water causes the body to produce something known as hormetic stress which activates pathways that help you to decrease sensitivity to stress and increase your stress tolerance. As stress can be a huge factor preventing sleep, this strategy could be worth exploring if relevant to you.

Beyond reducing stress, cold exposure can also help to alleviate anxiety. Cold stimulation, for example by placing ice on your chest and neck, can cause a shift in your parasympathetic nervous system (controlled by your vagus nerve, which oversees things like mood). This shift can help to slow down your heart rate and distract you from anxious thoughts and feelings that may be preventing you from sleeping well.

To practise cold exposure at home to reduce stress and anxiety and promote better sleep, you could experiment with cold showers or baths, washing your face in cold water, or drinking iced water.

Creating a sleep schedule or sleep goals

Our circadian rhythms can be very delicate, which is why having a consistent sleep schedule can be key to regaining control over your rest. When we get into a cycle of falling asleep around the same time each night and waking up around the same time each morning, it is easier for our bodies to stay in this rhythm. Our bodies look for patterns to follow, so when it comes to sleep, it is good to set yourself a goal for the number of hours' rest you desire.

Keeping a simple sleep schedule can help you to stay in control and get a clear idea of what other routines in your life may need to change to accommodate your goal. Data gives us objective insights into our habits and can help us connect cause and effect. While your current sleep habits could seem random, recording your personal sleep data (such as your current bedtimes, how many hours of sleep you get each night, etc.) over time can help you realize what aspects of your lifestyle could be responsible for your sleep issues.

Feel free to use the table provided on p.24 however works best for you. In the "Hours of Sleep" sections, you can either record the times you went to sleep and woke up, or simply the number of hours you slept or your energy level. By tracking your sleep habits, you can slowly understand your personal patterns and then make informed adjustments to improve your sleep.

	Hours of sleep	Energy Level		Hours of sleep	Energy Level
M		☆☆☆☆☆	M		☆☆☆☆☆
T		☆☆☆☆☆	T		☆☆☆☆☆
W		☆☆☆☆☆	W		☆☆☆☆☆
Th		☆☆☆☆☆	Th		☆☆☆☆☆
F		☆☆☆☆☆	F		☆☆☆☆☆
Sa		☆☆☆☆☆	Sa		☆☆☆☆☆
Su		☆☆☆☆☆	Su		

	Hours of sleep	Energy Level		Hours of sleep	Energy Level
M		☆☆☆☆☆	M		☆☆☆☆☆
T		☆☆☆☆☆	T		☆☆☆☆☆
W		☆☆☆☆☆	W		☆☆☆☆☆
Th		☆☆☆☆☆	Th		☆☆☆☆☆
F		☆☆☆☆☆	F		☆☆☆☆☆
Sa		☆☆☆☆☆	Sa		☆☆☆☆☆
Su		☆☆☆☆☆	Su		☆☆☆☆☆

Wrap your arms tightly round your body and, as you hold yourself, hold this one thought in your head: I've got you.

DOLLY ALDERTON
ON GETTING TO SLEEP

Physical activity can help

Being active both mentally and physically during the day can help you feel tired. Of course, if you are struggling with insomnia or another consistent sleep issue you may find yourself lacking the energy during the day to exercise. This can put you into a cycle where, due to inactivity, your body isn't physically tired at night, yet you wake up in the morning without the energy to exercise.

According to the World Health Organization's guidelines on Physical Activity and Sedentary Behaviour, there is evidence to suggest that physical activity is connected to improvements in sleep (as well as mental and cognitive health).

If you are struggling to find the energy to get back on track, try some of these simple activities. You can start with one activity a day, then slowly increase the intensity and time you spend exercising as you feel comfortable.

- A neighbourhood walk after dinner
- Dancing
- Stretching
- Swimming
- Yoga

Yoga poses and stretches for sleep

After a busy or stress-filled day, it can be hard to quieten our minds and slow down our bodies when we want to get into bed. Stress can leave us feeling jittery, antsy or shaky – all feelings that can prevent us from easily dozing.

Fortunately, there are yoga poses and stretches you can practise before bed to burn that residual energy from your day. Studies have shown that yoga can help you fall asleep faster and enhance the quality of your sleep as you sync the movements with your breath. Try some of the following poses, using your intuition and knowing your limits – do what feels good and calming for you.

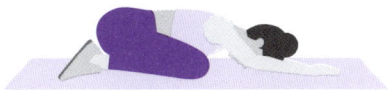
CHILD'S POSE

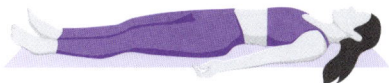
CORPSE POSE

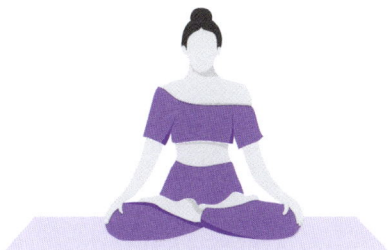
LOTUS POSE

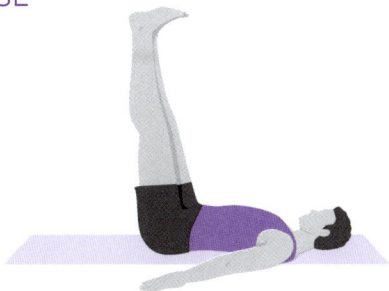
LEGS UP THE WALL POSE

SLEEP POSITIONS

The position we sleep in affects more than the quality of our rest. Do you wake yourself up with your own snoring or often feel tension in your neck or back in the mornings? If so, your sleep position could be the cause.

Ensuring that your spine is properly aligned while you're sleeping is key. This is easiest to achieve when sleeping on your side or back. While it is generally considered healthier to sleep in these two positions, sleeping on one's stomach can also be effective as long as you use the proper pillows and have a good mattress.

Side sleeping is particularly helpful in reducing heartburn and snoring, while sleeping on your back can prevent neck or back pain and reduce congestion. Pay attention to what position(s) you find most comfortable and, if your current sleeping position isn't working for you, try experimenting with another.

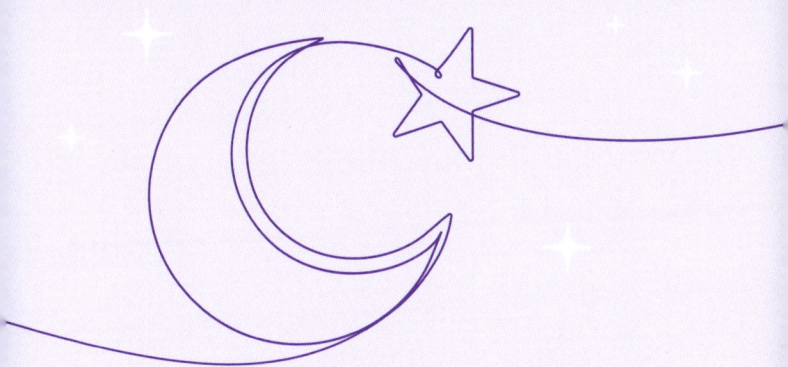

At the end of the day, I can end up just totally wacky, because I've made mountains out of molehills. With meditation, I can keep them as molehills.

RINGO STARR

Going to bed earlier

If you're tired of being tired all the time, it might seem obvious to go to sleep earlier. But it's hard to force this change overnight (if your bedtime is currently after 12.00 a.m., your body probably isn't tired at 9.30 p.m.). According to the ResMed Global Sleep Survey of 2024, nearly 40 per cent of participants get less than three nights of good sleep weekly and 50 per cent experience excessive daytime sleepiness.

Going to bed earlier can help improve feelings of restfulness but, to be effective, changing the time at which you go to bed should be done slowly and deliberately. Try going to sleep earlier in 30-minute increments until you've reached your desired bedtime. Getting into bed about an hour before you want to fall asleep can also be useful in changing your current sleep pattern, giving you time to unwind without the stress of striving to fall asleep instantly or at an exact time.

Before changing your bedtime, consider what aspects of your night-time routine you will also need to modify so they're done before you plan on going to sleep (having dinner, showering, skin care, getting into pyjamas, etc.).

CREATING COSINESS

Getting into bed under a soft duvet, wearing a T-shirt that's perfectly soft from a million washes, is of course going to feel cosier than crashing on the couch.

Explore these upgrades for extra cosiness:

- **Comforters:** If you're warm while you sleep, you will probably want a lightweight blanket made of a breathable fabric, whereas colder sleepers may want a heavier comforter.

- **Mattress:** Each mattress type has its own pros and cons, so consider things like your sleeping position to ensure your mattress best supports your body's specific needs.

- **Pillows:** Down and down-alternative pillows can be comfy while still supporting your head and neck.

- **Pyjamas:** Take time to ritualize changing into your pyjamas in the evening and choose fabrics that are comfortable for you. While cotton is a common favourite, linen and bamboo are other options. For those who feel cold in the evenings, wool and other heavy materials can be worth exploring.

- **Sheets and pillowcases:** Cotton and linen are breathable and often selected for sheets, but silk can be a wonderful choice for pillowcases as the material is great for your hair and skin.

DAILY CHORES

As previously discussed, decluttering your bedroom can be helpful for nurturing your sense of rest and relaxation.

Try to check these daily chores off your to-do list each morning:

- Make your bed
- Move things back to their designated places
- Clear away any mugs or cups you may have on your bedside table
- Place any clothes you plan on washing in a laundry basket
- Fold and put away any other clothes
- Throw away any rubbish

If you share a room, you can take turns doing these daily chores or encourage whoever you live with to try integrating these tasks into their morning routine so the space can be comfortable for everyone each evening.

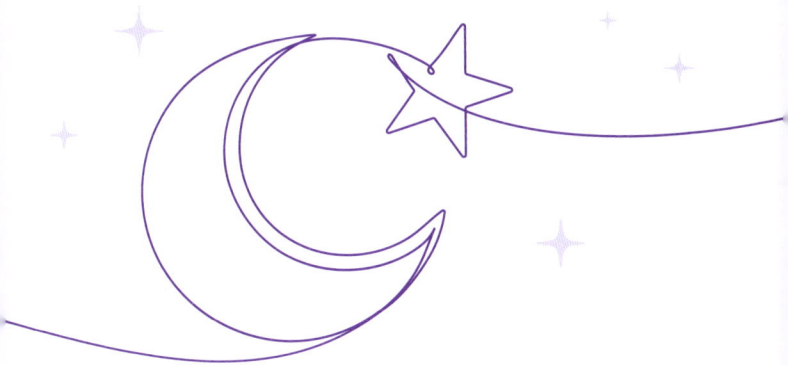

*Sleep is an investment
in the energy you need to
be effective tomorrow.*

TOM ROTH

Meditation

THE BASICS OF MEDITATION

Meditation is an ancient mindfulness practice that originated in India thousands of years ago. Associated with many religions (including Buddhism and Hinduism), meditation can be defined as a mental exercise with the purpose of reaching a heightened spiritual awareness. Similarly, mindfulness is the practice of maintaining a state of heightened awareness by paying close attention to your thoughts and surroundings. Meditation and mindfulness often go hand in hand.

Both mental exercises are highly adaptable and accessible – you can practise them in solitude or with others, at any time of day and anywhere that suits you. A lovely thing about meditation is that there is no right or wrong way to go about it. The practice is simply about learning techniques that help you clear your head. While various techniques are better for different outcomes, from reducing stress to strengthening empathy, every form of meditation can be modified to best support you and your goals.

In the following chapters, this book will guide you through various styles of meditation, allowing you to explore what is most effective for you. Although they vary, many styles of meditation integrate focused breathing, connecting with your thoughts and feelings, and freeing yourself from distractions.

With consistent practice, meditation and mindfulness should contribute to a feeling of calm you can return to at any time. For improving sleep, research suggests devoting 10–30 minutes a day to your practice.

TYPES OF MEDITATION AND THEIR BENEFITS

There are many different forms of meditation to explore. Using a variety of mental and physical techniques, ranging from contemplation and guided meditations to breathing exercises and mantras, meditation can help you relax, reduce anxiety and stress, and strengthen your ability to process emotions.

Using brain scans, researchers have been able to study the positive effects meditation has on the brain. Commonly, people who regularly meditate experience decreased anxiety, depression and PTSD, and improved focus.

There are so many techniques to choose from and it can take time to discover what works best for you – some of those listed below make an appearance in the following chapters, where you'll be able to put them into practice.

Types of meditation include:

- Body scan
- Chakra meditation
- Focused attention
- Guided meditation
- Loving-kindness
- Mantra meditation
- Mindfulness meditation
- Movement meditation
- Noting technique
- Progressive relaxation
- Resting awareness
- Skilful compassion
- Transcendental meditation
- Visualization
- Zen meditation

WHY MEDITATIONS CAN
HELP WITH SLEEP

Meditation is commonly known to improve mental and emotional well-being. However, looking at things holistically, it's important to recognize that our physical health is intrinsically linked to our mental and emotional states. Because of this connection, meditation also has the power to improve overall physical health, especially when it comes to sleep.

In the ResMed Annual Global Sleep Survey in 2023 – which collected information regarding sleep quality and habits from more than 20,000 people from 12 countries – anxiety and depression (along with work-related concerns) were among the most common reasons for lack of sleep, affecting 33 per cent of participants.

If you are struggling with sleep issues, integrating meditation into your routine could be a solution. Meditation targets the common issues of anxiety and depression, and by reducing or resolving any mental health struggles, can simultaneously improve your sleep. This is because meditation (especially methods that utilize breathing techniques) slows down your heart rate and helps lower the levels of cortisol (a stress hormone) in your body. These outcomes can reduce mental and emotional distress, while physically mimicking things the body naturally does while sleeping.

Learning about and experimenting with breathing techniques, mantras, visualizations and other meditation practices will allow you to connect with what works best for you and find tools you can tap into whenever you need a pause.

HOW TO PRACTISE
THESE MEDITATIONS

The following chapters will guide you through a series of meditations you can complete in 5, 10 or 15 minutes. Unless otherwise stated, they can be practised indoors or outside, at any time of day and in any position (including lying in bed), so long as your back is straight. With easy-to-follow directions, you may choose to read about an exercise and then try the technique on your own, or you can refer to the book during your meditation as you build up your confidence and intuition.

If you find yourself fixating on time, integrate setting a timer into any of the exercises. Additionally, feel free to have fun and explore combining some of the meditations and techniques such as music or aromatherapy with breathwork.

While specific recommendations are provided for each meditation regarding where, when and how to practise, remember that you can always do what feels comfortable for you. Although many of the exercises can be practised at any time of day, they are all designed with improving sleep in mind.

There are plenty of different styles of meditations to choose from – discovering which techniques benefit you the most can help you achieve a better night's sleep.

Put your thoughts
to sleep, do not let them
cast a shadow over
the moon of your heart.
Let go of thinking.

RUMI

CHAPTER TWO:

5-Minute
Meditations

MINDFUL BODY SCANNING

*Mindful body scanning is a form of
meditation in which you scan your body
for tension or emotional unease.*

TO PRACTISE:

1. Once you are lying down, begin by allowing your eyes to softly focus, staring at nothing in particular around you.

2. When you are ready, take a few deep breaths. As you slowly inhale through your nose, and exhale through your mouth, allow your eyes to close naturally as you move into a calm mental state.

3. With your eyes closed, begin by focusing on your head, noting if there is any tension present, and slowly move down through the rest of your body, ending with your toes.

4. You may repeat this process as many times as you need.

5. To soothe any feelings of tension, after your first body scan, you can restart and imagine warm sunshine moving down from your head to your toes as you rescan your body.

BREATHWORK

BOX BREATHING

There are lots of different breathing exercises that can be practised while meditating. Many forms of meditative breathing help calm the nervous system, reduce stress, enhance your immune system and increase your energy levels (which can be particularly helpful if you're struggling with sleep).

Box breathing is a specific breathing exercise that you can visualize as having four sides to it, like a box. Try practising this exercise before you go to bed. (It is commonly suggested that you don't exceed more than three to four rounds a couple of times a day.)

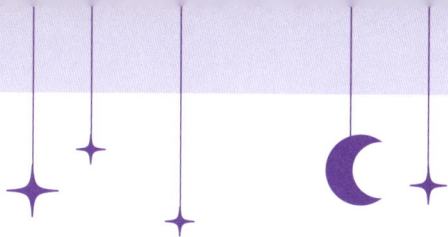

TO PRACTISE:

1. Get comfortable, breathing as you normally would and allowing your eyes to close naturally.

2. Whenever you're ready, start to consciously count the four-second intervals in your head, beginning by inhaling for four seconds.

3. Hold your breath for four seconds.

4. Exhale for four seconds.

5. Hold your breath again for four seconds and then repeat the whole process.

Box breathing helps lower stress, activates the parasympathetic nervous system (which affects rest and digestion) and brings you to a state of mindfulness.

If you're new to breathing exercises, it can be helpful to have one hand on your chest and one on your stomach so you can feel the connection between your breath and body as your chest and stomach rise with each inhale.

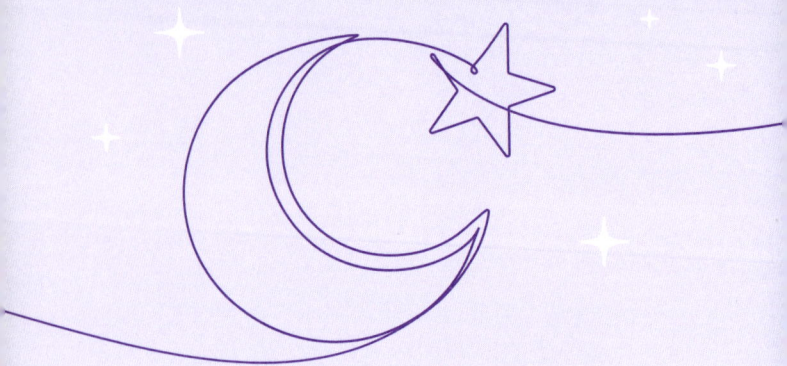

*It's very important that
we re-learn the art of
resting and relaxing.*

THÍCH NHẤT HẠNH

4-7-8 BREATHING

Another breathing meditation that is helpful for sleep is the 4-7-8 technique. This meditation can be practised seated, with good posture to support your back. It is commonly suggested that you don't exceed more than three to four rounds a couple of times a day.

TO PRACTISE:

1. Start by getting comfortable and breathe as you normally would.

2. You can either let your eyes softly focus on the space around you or allow them to close naturally.

3. When you're ready, inhale through your nose for four seconds.

4. Hold your breath to a count of seven.

5. Exhale through your mouth for eight seconds.

6. Then repeat the whole process – you can change the speed at which you count to four, seven and eight as long as you stay consistent with your pacing.

BREATH COUNTING MEDITATION

Similar to box breathing or the 4-7-8 technique, breath counting meditation is an exercise that can help you concentrate on your mind–body connection. It is perfectly acceptable (and natural) for the mind to wander while meditating. The beauty of a counting-based meditation is that it provides your mind with something specific to focus on.

TO PRACTISE:

1. Sit comfortably, with good posture to support your back.

2. Breathe as you normally would, allowing yourself to feel grounded wherever you're seated.

3. Once calm, begin to take deeper breaths, feeling your chest and stomach rise as you fully take in the air.

4. When your breathing feels comfortable, start to count your breaths as follows: inhale, hold, exhale one, inhale, hold, exhale two...

5. Continue until you've reached a count of ten.

If your mind wanders at any point and you lose track of what number you were on, simply start over at one.

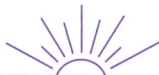

Variations: Once you feel comfortable and have gained enough focus to count your breaths to ten, you can also do the meditation reversed (counting backward from ten to one). You can also count to a higher number as you build your skills.

✦ ALTERNATE NOSTRIL BREATHING ✦

This yogic breathing technique helps to create balance in your breathing as you alternate between using just one nostril at a time. You can practise this while doing another meditation exercise to help you sleep.

TO PRACTISE:

1. Begin by sitting cross-legged, with good posture to support your back.

2. Focus on your breathing.

3. Have your left hand on your left knee and hold your right hand toward your nose.

4. Exhale fully and then close your right nostril with your finger.

5. Inhale through your left, open nostril.

6. Open your right nostril and close your left nostril with your finger.

7. Exhale through your right nostril.

8. Inhale through your right nostril.

9. Close your right nostril with your finger again, and exhale through your left nostril.

10. Inhale through your left nostril.

11. Repeat for five minutes and then finish the meditation by exhaling through your left nostril.

As you experiment, you can choose to hold your breath after each inhale for about two to three seconds before exhaling.

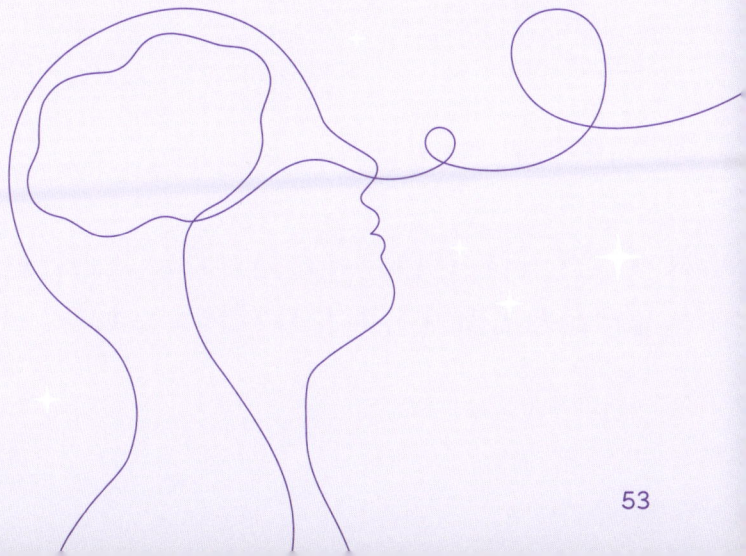

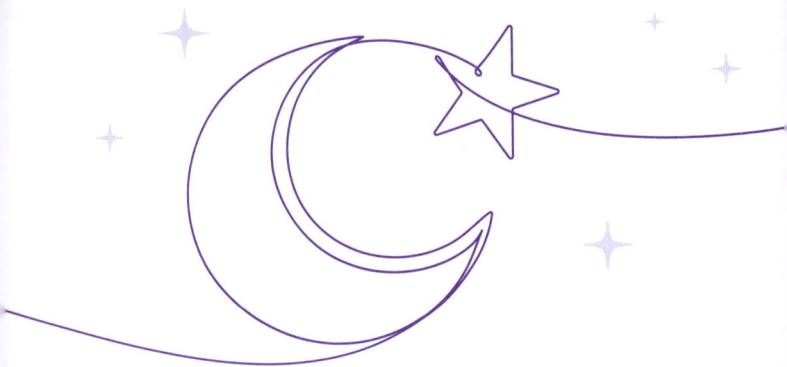

Within you, there is a stillness and a sanctuary to which you can retreat at any time and be yourself.

HERMANN HESSE

Buteyko breathing is designed to help breathlessness, anxiety and sleep issues by resetting and balancing your breathing. There are in-person training sessions to learn Buteyko breathing, but you can safely try it at home. The most important thing to keep in mind is to always inhale and exhale through your nose (not your mouth) when practising this technique.

TO PRACTISE:

1. Sit comfortably, with good posture to support your back.
2. Breathe normally through your nose with your mouth gently closed.
3. When you're ready, after an exhale, hold your breath.
4. Use your fingers to plug your nose.
5. When you feel like you need to inhale again, unplug your nose and breathe normally for at least ten seconds.
6. Again (when you're ready), after an exhale, hold your breath and plug your nose.
7. Repeat these steps.

SOUND

MUSIC MEDITATION

Did you know there's music designed to accompany meditation? From nature sounds to singing bowls, there are lots of options to choose from. Many researchers have found that music has a multitude of therapeutic effects – similar to meditation.

Incorporating music into your meditation practice can help you focus your attention on sound rather than the thoughts in your head, making this a great technique for beginners. By combining breathwork and music meditation, you can unlock another level of calm as you grow more comfortable with meditating. We'll explore music meditation further (see pp.142–3), but if you're looking to meditate for about five minutes, you can start with just a single song.

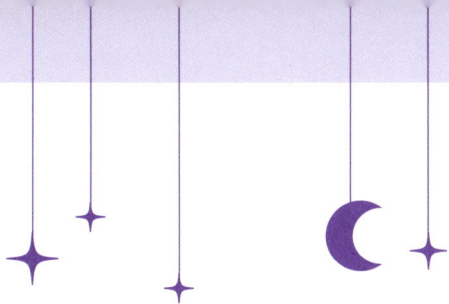

TO PRACTISE:

1. When choosing a song for this practice, consider if there's already a piece of music that makes you feel calm whenever you hear it. If you're not sure where to start, something classical, instrumental or ambient could be ideal.

2. Get comfortable and queue your chosen song (consider setting it to loop automatically so that you can continue to meditate longer if you find yourself getting into a flow state).

3. Click play when you're ready.

4. Follow the directions for any of the breathing exercises (see pp.46–55).

Just as in sleep our brains relax and give us dreams, so at some time in the day we need to disconnect, reconnect, and look around us.

LAURIE COLWIN

MANTRA MEDITATION

A mantra is a sound, word or phrase you repeat while meditating. Similar to counting meditations, mantras help focus your mind on the present. Repeating a word or phrase in your head or out loud can reduce brain activity which has a calming effect that's wonderful for sleep.

TO PRACTISE:

1. Lie down in bed on your back (or in a position that is most comfortable for you), softly focusing on the space around you.

2. Breathe normally and, when you're ready, close your eyes.

3. As you breathe, repeat a restful sound, word or phrase like "I am calm and ready to sleep" in your head or out loud, gently refocusing on your mantra should your mind wander.

AROMATHERAPY
MEDITATION

We've started exploring how sensory elements, like music or sound, can help to create a sense of calm and focus during meditation. Well, so can smell!

Our sense of smell is directly connected to the brain, making it very powerful. Scents set off electrical signals that are connected to the part of our brain associated with memory and emotions. Aromatherapy meditation allows you to form strong associations between certain smells and the calming feeling meditating produces, which can help you experience better sleep.

You may already have strong associations with particular smells. Whether it's the scent of a specific perfume or cologne, the beach, or something home-cooked, smells like these can help you to tap into various emotions. For aromatherapy meditation, you'll want to select a calming scent in the form of a room spray, incense or essential oil (which is particularly handy when you're on the move).

TO PRACTISE:

1. Prepare your chosen form of aromatherapy, either spraying the area, lighting the incense or adding a few drops of essential oil to a diffuser.

2. Follow the directions for any of the breathing exercises (see pp.46–55) or another meditation exercise of your choice.

Some well-known scents for sleep include frankincense and myrrh, lavender, neroli, vetiver and ylang-ylang. Do check the side effects for your essential oil of choice before you use it as some aren't suitable for certain people.

VISUALIZATION

Some people struggle with staying asleep due to nightmares. When things that are causing us stress are unresolved in the day, our minds often try to work through them when we're sleeping at night. While this can be useful, if you've ever woken up from a nightmare, you know the feeling is not one of restfulness!

Visualization is a meditation technique in which you use your imagination to create a mental image of a person, object, place or experience. This visual sensory work can be powerful because the brain has a hard time distinguishing between visualizations and the reality of the present moment. The technique also helps with neuroplasticity – the brain's ability to create new pathways, adapt and change – which allows you to more easily achieve what you're visualizing in real life.

TO PRACTISE:

1. Find somewhere comfortable to sit where you will be able to write in a journal.

2. Sit or recline with your materials ready (a journal and something to write with).

3. Focus on your breath.

4. As you inhale and exhale, bring your awareness to a sense of support from your bed, chair or the floor.

5. In a journal, write down a dream or dreams you'd like to have in as much detail as possible.

6. Once you've journalled, close your eyes and visualize your chosen dream with as much sensory detail as you can.

7. Allow this exercise to help you sleep peacefully and hopefully nightmare-free (you may also integrate music or aromatherapy – see pp.56–7 and 60–1).

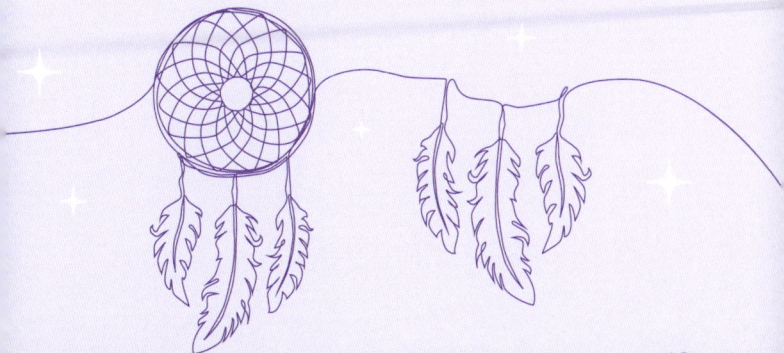

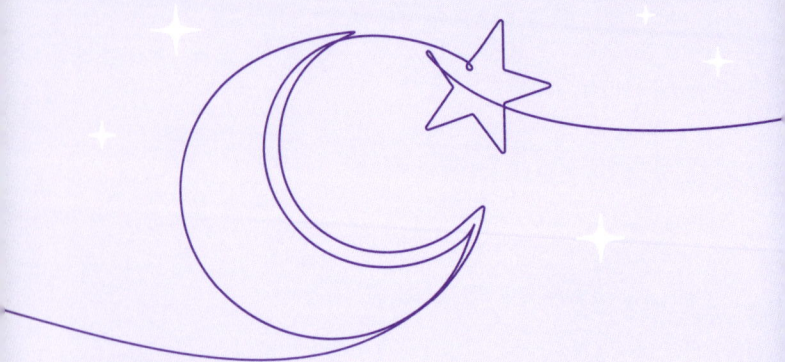

Real rest feels like every cell is thanking you for taking care of you.

JENNIFER WILLIAMSON

CLOUD MEDITATION

When we take the time to slow down and check in with ourselves, the thoughts in our heads can seem loud or overwhelming. This can be particularly annoying when you're trying to sleep – which is where cloud meditation comes in.

Rather than letting yourself hyperfixate on or investigate all your thoughts and feelings, you can visualize them as clouds drifting through the sky.

TO PRACTISE:

1. Lie in bed on your back (or in a position that is most comfortable for you) with your eyes closed.

2. As you breathe, let your mind wander as it wants (don't bother trying to control your thoughts).

3. When you're ready, begin to imagine each thought as a cloud and let each cloud drift from one side of the sky to the other until it's no longer in view.

4. Repeat this process until your imagined sky is cloudless, allowing you to drift off to sleep.

REMEMBERING YOUR BEST SLEEP

The possibilities for using visualization in your meditation practice are as unlimited as your own imagination. We've looked at creating mental images, but drawing from our memories is also powerful.

If you used to fall asleep easily, it can feel extra frustrating to go through a phase of insomnia or sleep issues. However, tapping into the memory of when you slept soundly can be the key to getting back on track.

TO PRACTISE:

1. Lie down in bed on your back (or in a position that is most comfortable for you) and close your eyes.

2. As you breathe, try to remember a time when you experienced wonderful sleep.

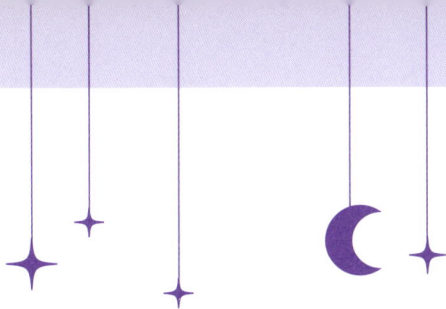

3. Once you remember this experience, try visualizing it in as much sensory detail as possible. (What did the bedding feel like? Could you hear things like rain, the wind or the ocean?).

4. As you visualize this sleeping experience, you can integrate mantras into your practice (see p.59) to tell yourself you will sleep as well as this again.

If you find this exercise helpful, take time to reflect on any differences between how you're currently sleeping and what you're visualizing. For example, if you're visualizing a bed with comfy pillows and yours are not, you may want to buy new ones. Or, if you're visualizing sleep on a beach vacation, you may want to start listening to ocean sounds as you sleep.

COLOUR MEDITATION

Colours have a range of different meanings in meditation and by visualizing them you can better understand or change your mental state.

TO PRACTISE:

1. Visualize a particular colour while doing breathwork (see pp.46–55) or use a particular colour while doing a drawing meditation (see pp.78–81).

2. Imagine the colour itself or imagine things of that colour – if you're thinking of green, for example, you may think of grass, seaweed and clover.

3. Alternatively, you can close your eyes, visualizing the colour you're currently feeling and focus on that colour transforming into the colour you'd like to be feeling (for helping with sleep, perhaps this colour would be blue as it's associated with calmness).

Some of the meanings behind various colours include:

- **Red:** balance, groundedness, love, passion, strength
- **Orange:** confidence, creativity, energy, power, relatability
- **Yellow:** happiness, inner power, intellect, logic, optimism, potential
- **Green:** compassion, enlightenment, forgiveness, inner peace, nature, self-acceptance, success, unconditional love
- **Blue:** calmness, communication, inner security, loyalty, open-mindedness, responsibility, self-expression, trust
- **Purple:** connection to higher consciousness, harmony of mind, inner imaginings, introspection, spirituality, wisdom
- **Pink:** romance, sensuality
- **Grey:** acceptance and understanding, neutrality
- **Brown:** earthiness, stability
- **Black:** protection from unwanted attention and criticism, sadness, secrecy
- **White:** intuition, pure energy, truth

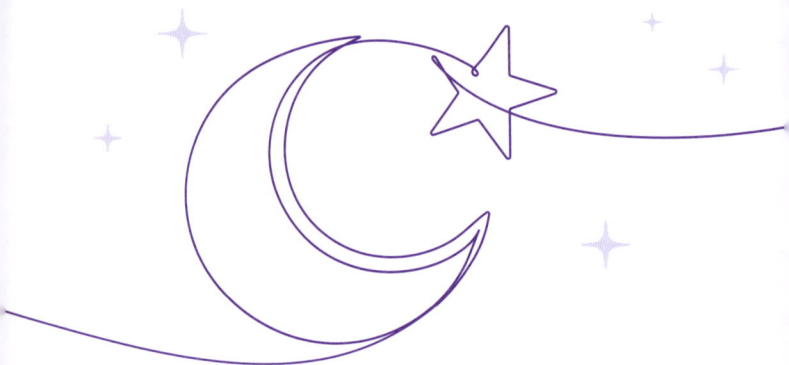

Meditation and praying
change your spirit into
something positive.

TINA TURNER

INNER CHILD MEDITATION

When we're struggling with sleep, or anything in life, it's easy to be hard on ourselves. However, this is not conducive to restfulness. Sleeping well requires gentleness and compassion, which can be hard to access after a long day. Next time you're having trouble falling asleep, rather than getting upset with yourself, try imagining yourself as a child. How would you treat the little kid you're imagining if they couldn't fall asleep? Would you sing them a song, read them a story... and maybe another story after that?

TO PRACTISE:

1. Lie down in bed on your back (or in a position that is most comfortable for you) and close your eyes.

2. Breathe slowly, imagining all the love and gentleness you'd provide for your child-self struggling to doze off.

3. While imagining this, wrap your arms around yourself in a hug.

WISH MEDITATION

When did you last check in with your inner child? If it's been a while, it can be hard to reconnect with the wants and needs of that version of yourself. Luckily, this wish meditation is designed to foster reconnection and soothe stress while helping you to fall asleep more easily.

This meditation is best done on a clear evening when you can see the moon and/or the stars.

TO PRACTISE:

1. Get comfortable outside or position yourself somewhere inside, facing a window. You can be in any position (including lying in bed), as long as your back is straight.

2. While breathing, look at the sky with a soft focus (you can keep your eyes open or eventually allow them to close gently if this is comfortable for you).

3. As you breathe, let your mind wander at first then slowly recall memories of wishing upon stars, eyelashes or birthday candles when you were younger – try remembering what you would wish for.

4. Think of something you'd like to wish for tonight (like rejuvenating sleep) then place a hand over your heart to connect the rise of your breath with your wish.

5. Continue to focus on your breathing – allow yourself to feel all the emotions of the wish you are putting out into the evening and know that, through reconnecting with the desires of your inner child, you can drift off into a calming and nurturing sleep.

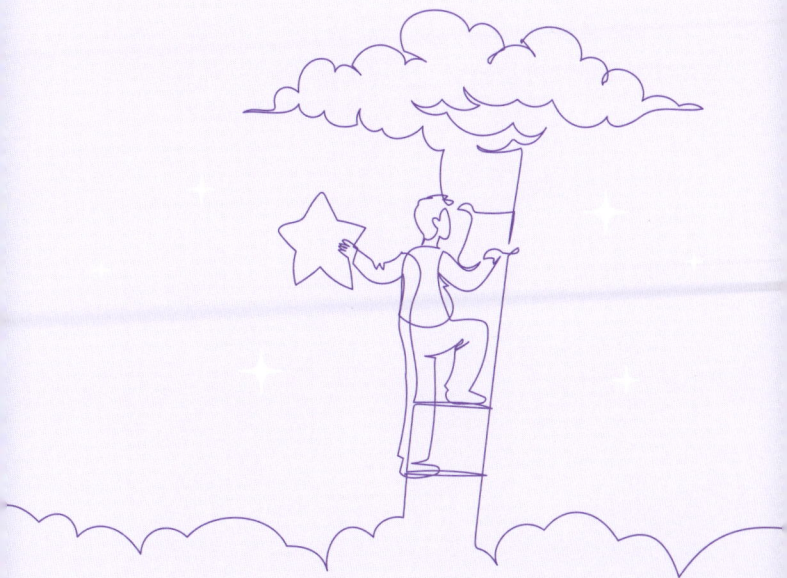

MANDALA MEDITATION

FOCUSING ON MANDALAS

Mandalas are sacred symbols (rooted in Buddhism and Hinduism) commonly used in meditation. Research shows that simply looking at mandalas can ease stress and depression, and help with sleep.

From videos to books full of these mesmerizing illustrations, there are many places in which to find mandalas to look at while meditating.

TO PRACTISE MEDITATION USING A MANDALA:

1. Sit comfortably on the floor, on a chair or in your bed.

2. Either use the illustrations on pp.75–6 (or on p.107), or look for a mandala that speaks to you.

3. Create an intention for your meditation (this can be as simple as "I'd like to sleep soundly").

4. When you're ready, focus on the mandala while inhaling and exhaling slowly.

5. Your eyes will probably be drawn to the centre of the mandala, moving outward as you take in the design – there's no "right" way to do this, so simply let your eyes guide your focus.

6. If your mind wanders, gently refocus on the mandala and the intention you set for this meditation.

7. Complete your meditation by calmly inhaling through your nose and exhaling through your mouth.

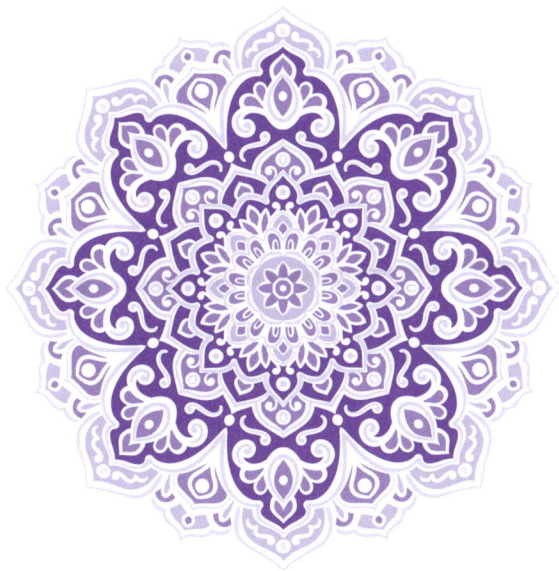

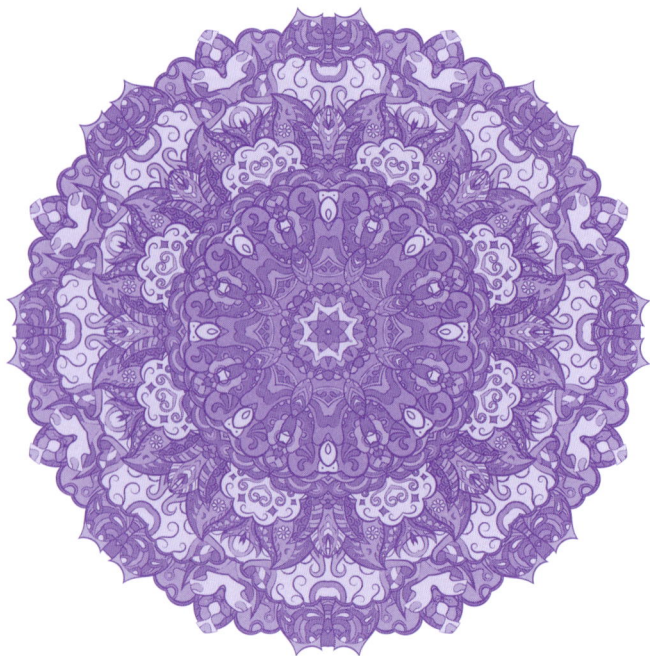

Almost everything will work again if you unplug it for a few minutes, including you.

ANNE LAMOTT

DRAWING THE
BREATH MEDITATION

*Drawing the breath, as the name suggests,
is a mindfulness exercise that involves
you literally drawing your breath! This
technique is especially accessible to beginners
because, while many meditation practises
are very inward-focused, drawing the breath
gives you something to do outwardly.*

TO PRACTISE:

1. Find a place where you will be comfortable to sit and draw.

2. Sit down with some paper and something to draw with.

3. As you breathe, allow your hand to move intuitively with your breath on the paper, creating various lines, shapes and patterns (if you want more guidance to begin, place your pencil on the centre of the left-hand side of your paper, draw a line upward as you

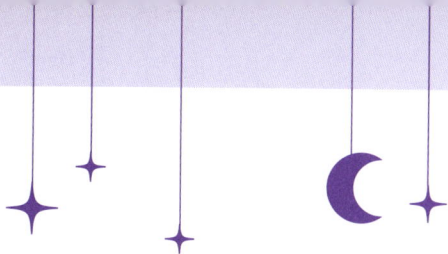

inhale, pause, and then continue the line, curving downward as you exhale).

4. Observe what happens when your breath is faster or slower – when stressed and breathing quickly you may draw in a chaotic way, but when calm and breathing slowly you might draw more smoothly.

5. Continue to inhale and exhale, fully and slowly.

6. Carry on drawing in a way that captures this focused breathing, emulating the sort of relaxed inhales and exhales you'd associate with sleep and restfulness until you feel calm or ready for bed.

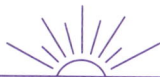

Variation: You can combine this practice with colour meditation (see pp.68–9) by using a specific colour connected with your intention.

REVERSE DRAWING THE BREATH MEDITATION

Drawing the breath is a great creative exercise for strengthening the mind–body connection and, as with all meditation practices, it can also help with improving sleep. You can also reverse this technique to influence your breathing. If you're hyperventilating or struggling to slow down your breathing, this method can help.

TO PRACTISE:

1. Find a place where you will be comfortable to sit and draw.

2. Sit down with some paper and something to draw with.

3. As you breathe, draw lines, shapes and patterns that you feel represent breathing slowly and calmly.

4. See how your breath is influenced by, and tries to match the movement of, your hand as you draw.

5. Continue drawing in a way that captures your desired breathing.

6. Complete this practice when your breath feels in tune with your drawing.

If this practice (both the regular and reversed version) resonates, it can be helpful to keep your drawings to observe how they change over time (hopefully, with practice, representing calmer breathing). You can even record on the back of the paper the date of each meditation, any feelings or thoughts about the experience, and updates on things like your sleep and overall well-being.

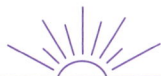

Variation: You can combine this practice with colour meditation (see pp.68–9) by using a specific colour connected with your intention.

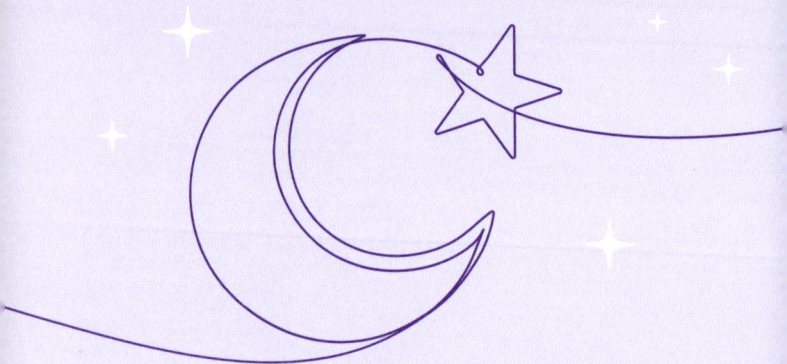

Insomnia is a glamorous
term for thoughts you
forgot to have in the day.

ALAIN DE BOTTON

It's a lifelong gift.
It's something you can
call on at any time.

PAUL McCARTNEY
ON MEDITATION

CHAPTER THREE:

10-Minute Meditations

BREATHWORK

COUNTING 100 BREATHS MEDITATION

While comparable to other breathwork-based meditation, counting 100 breaths offers an opportunity to bring your focus onto your breath for a longer period, which can be helpful for falling asleep or getting back to sleep if you wake up.

TO PRACTISE:

1. Sit or lie down with your hands resting on your lap or legs.

2. Your eyes can be open with a soft focus on the space around you (or closed if you're trying to fall asleep).

3. Allow yourself to breathe normally and, when you're ready, begin at 100, and count backward in your head with each exhale.

4. Your mind may wander and that is okay – if you lose count, simply begin again, allowing yourself to become more relaxed as you meditate or fall asleep.

JOURNALLING MEDITATION

Often, specific stressors like financial pressures or interpersonal issues prevent us from falling asleep. It makes perfect sense that when we're busy all day, these worries can feel louder around bedtime.

Journalling is a mindfulness activity that can help you meditate, freeing mental space so you can focus on your breath and relaxation. Rather than ignoring stressful thoughts, this meditation can help you acknowledge night-time worries and create space for you to return to them at a time that is convenient for you.

TO PRACTISE:

1. Find somewhere comfortable to sit where you will be able to write in a journal.
2. Sit or recline with your materials ready (a journal and something to write with).
3. Close your eyes and focus on your breathing.

4. As your mind slows down with your breath, simply act as an observer, seeing what thoughts come up as your mind naturally wanders.

5. When you feel ready, open your eyes and make a list in your journal of anything that is causing you stress.

6. Whether there's one thing or several, come up with a convenient time to brainstorm solutions for each item (for example, if you're having issues with a co-worker, worrying about this before bed is not exactly helpful; instead, perhaps this issue could have space at 10.00 a.m. on Friday).

7. While writing, visualize the worry or stress moving from your brain into your journal.

8. When done, close your eyes again to round out this meditation with additional focused breathing.

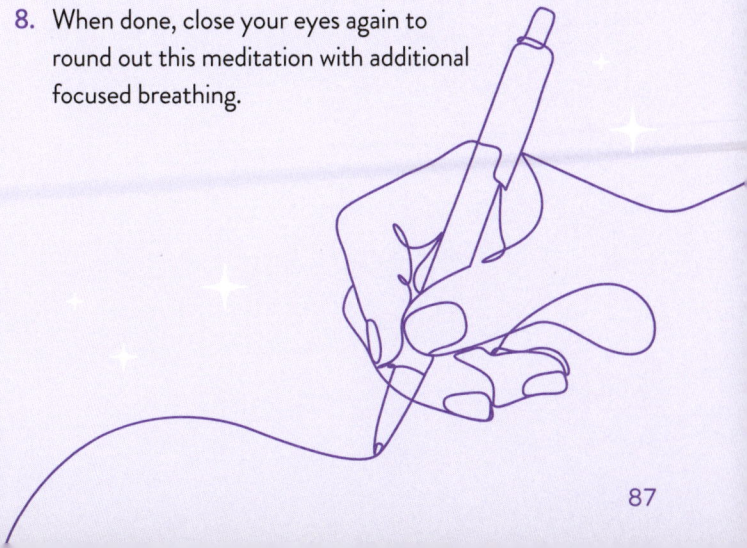

RELATIONSHIPS

Sometimes, in the evenings, you may find yourself ruminating on relationship struggles in your life. Whether you're worried about your connections with friends, family or romantic partners, these concerns can easily prevent you from falling asleep.

In this meditation, you will use a journal to reflect on any relationships causing you stress with a loving-kindness technique (a type of meditation that focuses on generating love, kindness and compassion for yourself and/or others).

TO PRACTISE:

1. Find somewhere comfortable to sit where you will be able to write in a journal.

2. Sit or recline with your materials ready (a journal and something to write with).

3. Begin by writing down the name of someone you are facing challenges with and any details you wish to add.

4. Once you're done journalling, close your eyes and focus on your breathing.

5. Call to mind the image of the person you wrote about, remembering they are a human just like you.

6. Try to imagine surrounding that person with love and kindness.

7. Visualize compassion for them radiating from their heart like rays from the sun.

8. Continuing to breathe calmly, imagine that those rays are warming you with love, kindness and compassion, allowing you to release conflict and drift off to sleep.

3-3-3

Research suggests that having a journalling practice supports better mental and physical health (as well as sleep quality). Journalling complements meditation as both practices allow us to slow down, acknowledging and reflecting on our thoughts and feelings without judgement.

This 3-3-3 journalling meditation provides you with the space to reflect on your day while also setting intentions.

TO PRACTISE:

1. In the evening, find somewhere comfortable to sit where you will be able to write in a journal.
2. Sit or recline with your materials ready (a journal and something to write with).
3. Close your eyes and focus on your breathing for a few minutes while reflecting on your day.

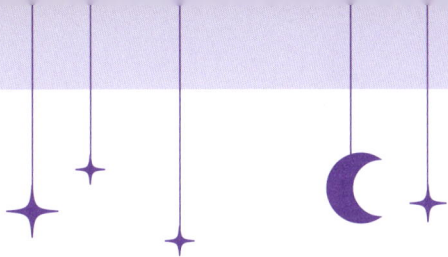

4. Simply observe the feelings or memories that wander through your mind as you take this time for yourself to slow down.

5. When you're ready, open your eyes and open your journal to a blank page.

6. Write down three things that brought you joy today, three things that are causing you stress and three intentions for yourself (such as getting a good night's sleep).

7. Once you're done journalling, close your eyes again and focus on your new intentions – try to fully embody what it would feel like if everything you're hoping for were your reality.

8. As you complete this particular meditation, remember that you've done the work of acknowledging your stress (rather than forcing your worries away when you're trying to rest) and have energetically brought yourself closer to your intentions.

SENSORY MEDITATION

Just as we've discussed how various stimuli like music and visual art can be integrated into meditations to enhance focus, we can also use our own senses for the same purpose.

Sensory meditation is about using our five senses – sight, smell, sound, taste and touch – to bring us heightened awareness of the present while aiding in stress relief and emotional regulation.

TO PRACTISE:

1. Stand, sit, or recline with your back straight, inhaling and exhaling peacefully.

2. As you breathe, move through each of your senses, beginning with sight.

3. With a soft focus, look at the space around you.

4. Closing your eyes, move your focus to your nose and ask yourself what you can smell.

5. Then, take notice of any sounds, tuning in to what you can hear.

6. Bring your attention to your mouth and consider what you can taste.

7. Continue observing your senses without judgement and, finally, consider what you can touch (What are the physical feelings in your own body? What does the surface beneath you feel like? What textures can you feel with your hands?).

8. Let your mind wander as you continue to breathe slowly, ending this practice feeling calm and restful.

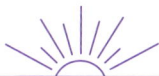

Variation: You can focus on the senses in any order, focus on fewer senses, or try to observe the same number of things for each sense.

A good laugh and a long sleep are the two best cures for anything.

IRISH PROVERB

VISUALIZATION

FREE FROM STRESS

Visualization meditations allow you to use your imagination to create a mental image of a person, object, place or experience. When stressors or worries are keeping you up at night, practising this free-from-stress visualization can help you fall asleep.

TO PRACTISE:

1. Get comfortable in bed, lying on your back (or in a position that is most comfortable for you).

2. Close your eyes, inhale through your nose and exhale through your mouth.

3. After a few focused breaths, breathe normally and imagine the things that are stressing you out as ice cream, snow, ice or another cold thing that resonates with you.

4. Allow your mind to interact with these visualizations.

5. Now, imagine the sun warming your stress until it melts away – can you feel the warmth on your skin? How does it feel to watch these visualizations slowly dissolve?

6. Complete this meditation by focusing on your breath.

✦ NOTING ✦

Noting is a common technique in which you mentally label your thoughts as thoughts and feelings as feelings. You can combine noting with almost any other exercise to strengthen introspectiveness and mindfulness, and gain the benefits of meditation (including improved sleep).

TO PRACTISE:

1. Stand, sit or recline in a position that is comfortable for you.

2. Begin by focusing on your breathing.

3. If your mind wanders, start to use noting – when a thought distracts you, simply label it as "thinking", using a calm inner voice; when a feeling distracts you, gently label it as "feeling".

4. Don't worry about noting everything – allow thoughts and feelings to pass and use noting when you get overly caught up in them.

5. Continue to focus on your breath and use noting any time you need to regain focus.

Noting is all about mental acknowledgement, letting go and moving on. By distilling your distractions down to a simple word, you can avoid spiralling and becoming preoccupied with where your mind wanders off to. It can be liberating to detach yourself from undesirable thoughts or feelings by labelling them, reminding yourself that that's all they are, and letting them go.

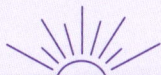

Variation: You can experiment by trying other labels like "worry", "daydream" or "future-thinking" that could better reflect where you find your mind wandering.

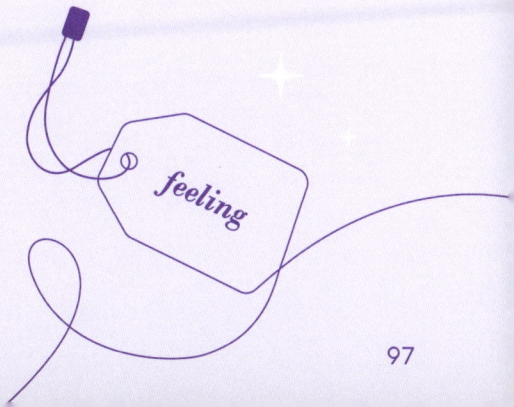

feeling

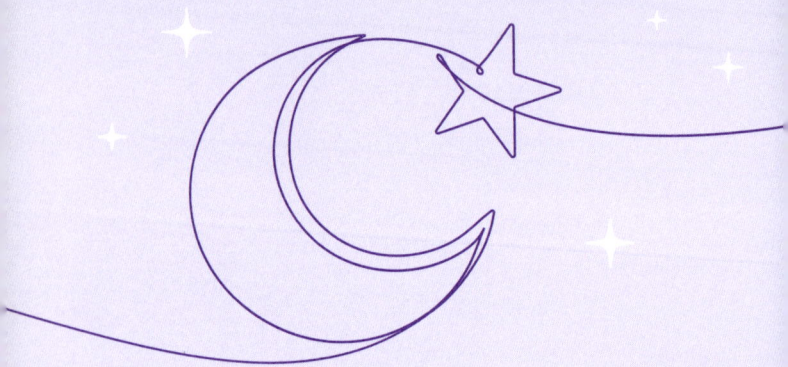

Having peace, happiness and healthiness is my definition of beauty. And you can't have any of that without sleep.

BEYONCÉ

INTERVAL TIMER MEDITATION

You can find free interval timer videos online that are specially designed to accompany meditation. These timers play calming sounds in set intervals, freeing you from worrying about how long you've been meditating or getting distracted by time.

TO INCORPORATE THIS TOOL INTO YOUR PRACTICE:

1. Get into a comfortable position, with your interval timer to hand.

2. Take a few deep breaths, inhaling through your nose and exhaling through your mouth to ground yourself before clicking play.

3. As you begin to meditate, allow your breath to return to its normal flow as you slowly close your eyes.

4. A calming sound (like a bell) will chime at a set interval.

5. Continue meditating in your desired style until you've reached ten minutes.

SOUND

SINGING BOWL MEDITATION

Singing bowls are tools you can use in your meditation practice to alleviate anxiety and improve well-being.

Sound healing and sound-based meditations have been used for centuries – singing bowls are simply another form, similar to music meditation (see p.56).

You can either use a singing bowl or a singing bowl video or playlist (available online and on music streaming platforms).

TO PRACTISE THIS STYLE OF MEDITATION:

1. Get into a comfortable position with your singing bowl, video or playlist to hand.

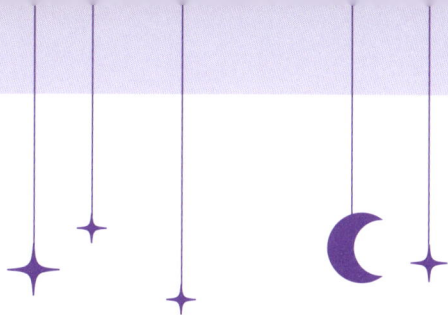

2. Take a few deep breaths while setting an intention for your meditation.

3. Click play on your singing bowl video or playlist or, if you have your own bowl, sit with your back straight and begin to chime your bowl, then swirl the striker around the outer edge to create a singing sound.

4. Whether you're listening to a recording or using a bowl, the sound should amplify over time – as it does, continue to focus on your breathing as you meditate, allowing the sound to increase your awareness and focus.

5. When you're ready to stop meditating, allow the video or playlist you've chosen to end or gradually slow down your circling of the bowl with the striker.

6. Sit or lie in silence for a few moments to reground yourself in your surroundings.

MALA BEAD MEDITATION

MANTRAS

Prayer and meditation beads, such as mala which originated in India, are centuries old and commonly used today for yoga and meditation. While there are variations, mala traditionally have 108 beads and a guru bead (which is bigger and usually has a tassel). When shopping for mala, you'll notice they come in a variety of materials and kinds of stones. Feel free to choose one with colours or a meaning that resonates with you.

Mala beads can complement mantra meditations (see p.59), helping you keep track of each repetition while enhancing focus, reducing stress, improving sleep and supporting your well-being.

TO COMBINE MALA BEADS WITH MANTRA MEDITATION:

1. Sit on the floor with your back straight and with your eyes closed or open (with a soft focus).

2. Set your intention for this practice and choose your mantra (anything from *om* to an affirmation of your choosing will work).

3. Slow down your breathing and hold your mala with the beads draping over your hand.

4. Place two fingers around one of the beads next to the guru bead and say, whisper or think your mantra to yourself.

5. Move on to the next bead and do the same, repeating for ten minutes or until you've reached the guru bead again (to do another round, simply reverse the direction).

After each practice, place your mala somewhere that is special to you so they'll have good energy for your next meditation.

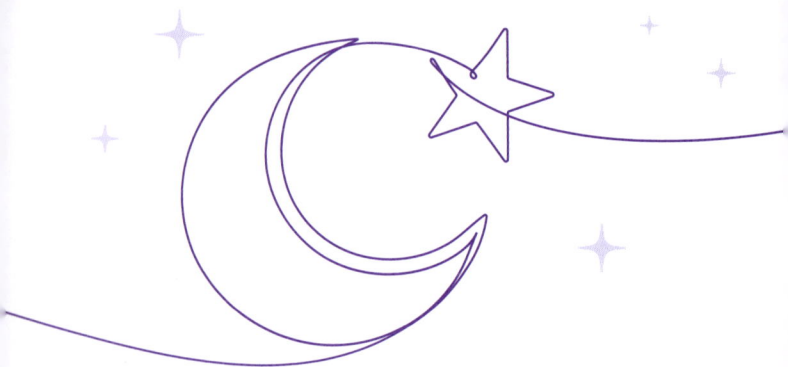

Finish each day before you begin the next, and interpose a solid wall of sleep between the two.

RALPH WALDO EMERSON

✦ COUNTING THE BREATH ✦

Mala beads can be useful alongside mantra-based meditations. They also complement breathwork and counting the breath styles of meditation (see pp.46–55).

TO USE MALA BEADS DURING A COUNTING THE BREATH MEDITATION:

1. Sit on the floor with your back straight and with your eyes closed or open (with a soft focus).

2. Slow down your breathing and hold your mala with the beads draping over your hand.

3. Place two fingers around one of the beads next to the guru bead.

4. Complete one full breath, inhaling and exhaling, then move your fingers to the next bead.

5. Repeat for ten minutes or until you've reached the guru bead again (to do another round, simply reverse the direction).

When you're done, place your mala somewhere that is special to you to keep them full of loving, calming energy.

MANDALA MEDITATION

COLOURING

Beyond looking at mandalas while setting intentions or practising breathwork (see pp. 74–6), colouring them in is also a type of meditation. Colouring in these intricate designs eases stress while providing an opportunity to connect with your sense of creativity and innovation.

TO PRACTISE THIS MEDITATION:

1. Find a place where you will be comfortable to sit and colour.

2. Sit with your colouring materials and this book.

3. Close your eyes and take a few deep breaths, setting your intentions for this meditation.

4. After meditating as you usually would, open your eyes and begin to colour in the mandalas here (there are more on pp.75–6, but you can also print illustrations or find colouring books).

5. As you're colouring, notice the way your breath naturally slows down, allowing you to focus on the present moment

– reflect on how it makes you feel to act intuitively, selecting the colours you gravitate toward.

6. When you have finished colouring in a mandala, look at it with a soft focus before closing your eyes to complete the meditation with a few more deep breaths – inhaling through your nose, and exhaling through your mouth.

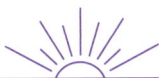

Variation: You can combine this practice with colour meditation (see pp.68–9) by drawing with specific colours connected to your intentions.

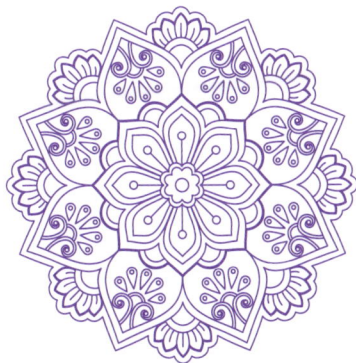

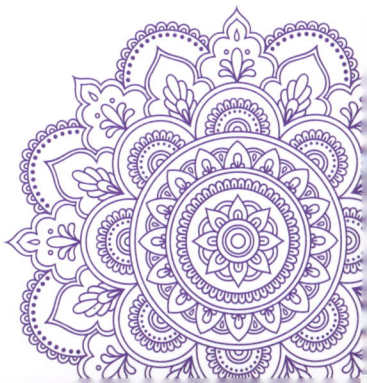

There is only one
thing people like that
is good for them:
a good night's sleep.

EDGAR WATSON HOWE

GUIDED MEDITATIONS

Guided meditations have been found to improve sleep – listening to calming stories and following someone else's words can shift your focus, allowing your mind to slow down as you drift off.

In preparation for your practice, choose a 10-minute guided meditation. These can be found online or on a music streaming platform. (While there are many for sleep, there are also guided meditations for other intentions with varying durations.)

TO PRACTISE:

1. With your guided meditation to hand, lie down in bed on your back (or in a position that is most comfortable for you).

2. Take a few deep breaths, inhaling through your nose and exhaling through your mouth. Click play on your guided meditation, gently close your eyes, and open your ears to follow along with the audio.

JAPA MEDITATION

Japa is a specific type of mantra or chanting meditation (see p.59) that originated in India. It reduces stress, calms the mind, activates various brainwaves, helps with focus, improves sleep and increases creativity. Mantra options are limited within Japa meditation and include om, so'hum *(meaning "I am that") and* om shanti shanti shanti *(pronounced "shaan-tee" and representing peace of body, mind and speech). Japa meditation is all about sticking with the same mantra every time you practise so, after experimenting, choose one that resonates with you. The meditation can be practised before sunrise, at sunset or at noon, and while walking, lying down or sitting on the floor.*

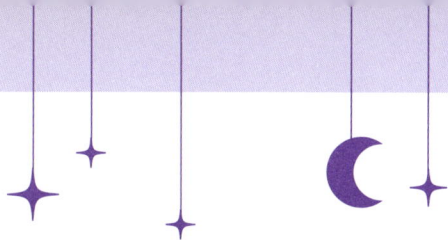

TO PRACTISE:

1. Partially close your eyes and maintain a soft focus.

2. Set intentions for your practice.

3. Choose a mantra: *om* is very powerful; however, some people like *so'hum* to help with focus (inhaling on *so* and exhaling on *hum*).

4. While breathing, repeat your mantra aloud (known as Vaikhari Japa), whispering (known as Upamanshu Japa), mentally (known as Manasika Japa) or by writing the mantra in a specially designed book while chanting aloud (known as Likhita Japa).

5. Complete your meditation with a few deep breaths – inhaling through your nose and exhaling through your mouth.

If you enjoy Japa meditation, consider incorporating mala beads to enhance focus further and keep track of your repetitions (see pp.102–3).

SHOWER MEDITATION

Shower meditation (also known as waterfall meditation) is a mindfulness practice that uses temperature and sound to stimulate your senses while improving focus, strengthening your mind–body connection and enhancing sleep.

Whether you're busy or feel like you're lacking space for solitude, shower meditation can be a great way to maintain or start a consistent meditation practice. Water cleanses the body and mind, and there's no right or wrong way to practise — simply allowing yourself to be present while you're showering has benefits.

TO PRACTISE:

1. Before showering, feel free to dim the lights, play music (see pp.56–7), or incorporate aromatherapy (see pp.60–1) to connect with the intentions you set for this practice.

2. Once you are in the shower (either standing or sitting), focus on your breathing.

3. Close your eyes and engage your senses as you inhale and exhale (What does the water feel like? Is it hot or cold? What does it sound like? What can you smell?).

4. Beginning with your head and working your way down to your toes, use visualization techniques to imagine the water washing away the day while physically cleansing your body of any emotional or mental burdens; imagine yourself inhaling calmness and exhaling negativity, letting it swirl down the drain with the water.

5. Complete your meditation by reflecting on your gratitude and breathing.

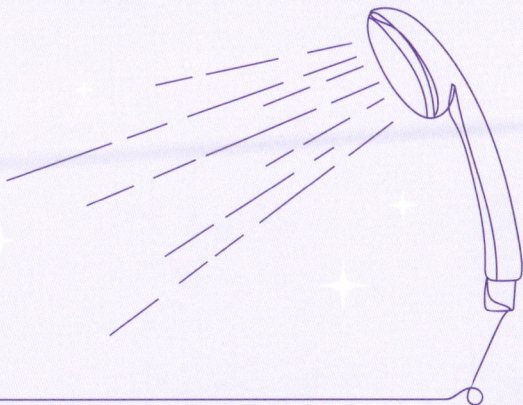

BATH MEDITATION

*Similar to shower meditation,
bath meditation engages your senses
to improve your focus, mind–
body connection and sleep.*

*Both shower and bath meditations are
great, especially for beginners, because
you are incorporating meditation into
an existing habit that involves self-care
in solitude. As with shower meditation,
there is no right or wrong when it comes
to meditating in the bath – simply
allow yourself to be present and calm.*

*For helping with sleep, this meditation
is best practised in the evening.*

TO PRACTISE:

1. As the bath runs, allow yourself to become mesmerized by the sight of the water falling from the tap, listen to the sound of the water running and use your sense of touch to appreciate the rising water level.

2. Once the bath is ready, feel free to dim the lights, play music (see pp.56–7) and/or incorporate aromatherapy (see pp.60–1) for a complete sensory experience.

3. Slowly lower yourself into the bath while focusing on your breathing.

4. Close your eyes and bring your awareness to what you can sense around you.

5. Use visualization techniques to imagine the water is embracing you in a hug or that the water is transforming any negative energy from your day into warmth and joy.

6. When you are ready to drain the water, continue meditating, visualizing any negativity swirling down the drain.

7. Complete your meditation by reflecting on your gratitude and breathing.

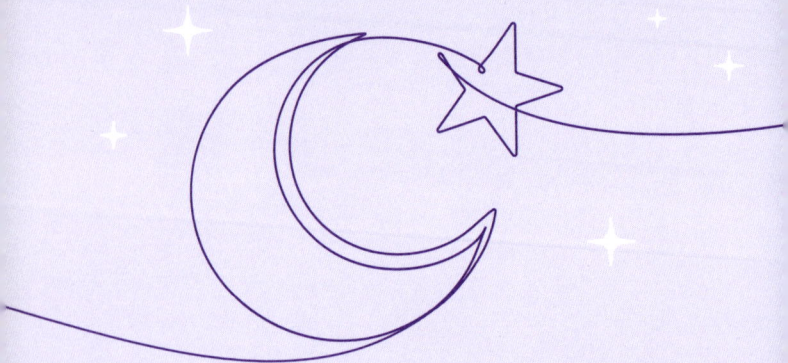

Tired minds don't plan well.
Sleep first, plan later.

WALTER REISCH

I love sleep because
it is both pleasant
and safe to use.

FRAN LEBOWITZ

PYJAMA MEDITATION

While this task may only take you a minute or two, extending the amount of time you take to get changed into comfortable clothes for bed can be an opportunity to practise mindfulness.

Using some of the techniques of mindful body scanning (see p.45), putting on your pyjamas can become an easy way to check in with yourself from head to toe, incorporating meditation into your bedtime.

TO PRACTISE PYJAMA MEDITATION:

1. Select your pyjamas with care while bringing awareness to your breath.

2. As you inhale through your nose and exhale through your mouth, begin mindful body scanning – start at your head, scanning for any stress.

3. Take your time to mentally move down through the rest of your body, inhaling sleepiness and exhaling stress as you put your pyjamas on in the same order you are scanning your body (as you start with your top and work down, observe the warmth and cosiness of the material).

4. Get comfortable in your bed and close your eyes.

5. Continue to focus on your breathing and scan your body again.

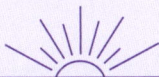

Variation: You can follow these same steps to meditate while getting dressed for your day as well.

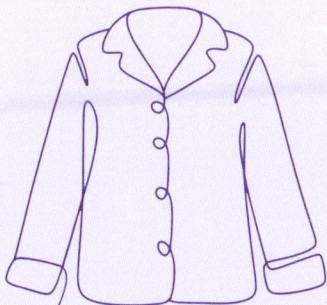

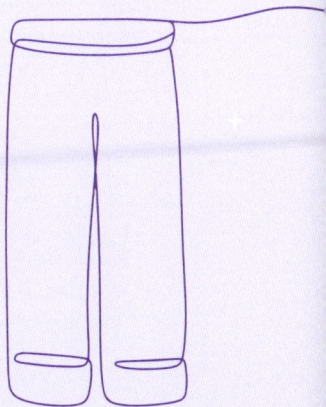

DO NOTHING MEDITATION

While guided meditations and breathwork exercises are incredibly helpful, sometimes it's good to just sit with your thoughts and feelings without directions. This free time and space is a great way to check in with yourself and hear your inner voice.

TO PRACTISE:

1. Set a timer for ten minutes.
2. In any position you choose, simply be – you can breathe normally, think about your day, get distracted, close your eyes, open your eyes; there is no right or wrong.
3. There's no need to do anything except be with yourself in your solitude until the timer goes off.

If you struggle with a racing mind before bed, this meditation provides space in your day for your wandering thoughts so you can experience improved sleep.

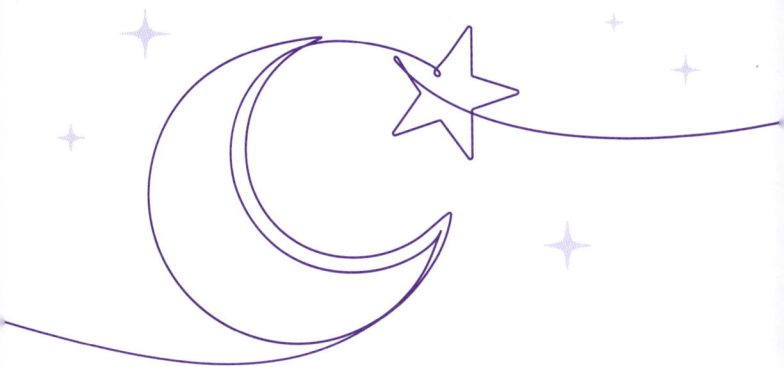

There is renewal in rest.

LAILAH GIFTY AKITA

CHAPTER FOUR:

15-Minute Meditations

FINANCE-BASED MEDITATION

Financial stress is one of the most common obstacles to sleep for many people. This meditation can help you to manage your feelings and thoughts, improve your focus and enhance your problem-solving skills.

TO PRACTISE:

1. Lie down in bed on your back.

2. Close your eyes, inhale through your nose and exhale through your mouth.

3. Scan your body (see p.45) for any stress and tune your attention inward.

4. Allow yourself to breathe naturally and bring to mind your specific worry or challenge.

5. Consider your relationship to and beliefs around money. (Do you often experience scarcity?)

6. Reflect on how you feel when you spend, save, earn, invest and give money.

7. Regardless of how you currently feel, imagine stability, fortune or peacefulness.

8. Refocus on the breath and imagine that what you have in this moment is enough.

TEA MEDITATION

A warm drink can be comforting and delightful, and research has shown that many teas can improve your rest and combat insomnia. So, why not combine tea with meditation?

For helping with sleep, this meditation is best practised in the evening.

TO PRACTISE:

1. Incorporate gratitude, intentionality and mindfulness into each step of the tea-making process, beginning by thoughtfully selecting a tea – green, chamomile, lavender, rose, jasmine and passionflower teas help with relaxation and lowering stress – and a mug.

2. Set the water to boil and focus on breathing and the sound of bubbling water as you wait.

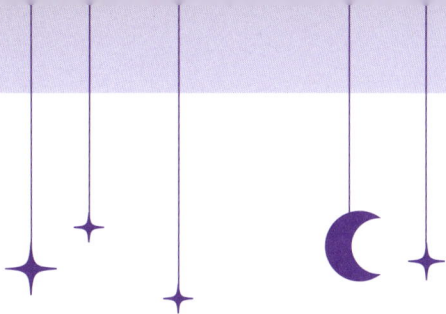

3. Pour the water into your mug, and observe the colour change as your tea steeps.

4. The aromas of certain teas (before consumption) have been found to help with mood – as the steam rises, close your eyes, inhale the smell of the tea through your nose and exhale through your mouth.

5. Building on the sensory experience, wrap your hands around the mug to feel the warmth, meditating as your tea cools.

6. When the tea is drinkable, inhale the smell, take a sip (savouring the flavour), swallow and exhale.

7. Continue this cycle or, if tired, set down your tea, gently close your eyes and focus on your breathing.

CHOCOLATE MEDITATION

In a similar way to tea meditation, you can create a mindful sensory experience for yourself using chocolate. Chocolate meditation has both neurological and psychological benefits (including reduced stress and improved sleep). Incorporating chocolate into your meditation practice gives you something to focus on while engaging your senses.

For helping with sleep, this meditation is best practised in the evening.

TO PRACTISE:

1. Incorporate gratitude, intentionality and mindfulness into each step of the process, beginning by thoughtfully selecting a chocolate – dark chocolate can lower blood pressure while cacao can help release mood-boosting chemicals like serotonin and tryptophan.

2. Sit or stand in solitude and take a few deep breaths – inhaling through your nose and exhaling through your mouth.

3. Continue focusing on your breathing as you observe everything from the way the chocolate feels in your hand to its smell, before closing your eyes and placing a small piece in your mouth.

4. Allow the chocolate to slowly melt on your tongue – mindful eating is about savouring the flavour of your food and taking time to appreciate the full sensory experience (seeing, smelling, hearing, tasting and feeling).

5. If your mind wanders, gently guide your thoughts back to the chocolate.

6. You may repeat this process as desired.

7. When done, take a few more deeps breaths to complete this meditation.

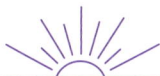

Variation: If chocolate isn't for you, feel free to use another treat that can melt in your mouth.

MINDFUL EATING MEDITATION

Chocolate meditation is simply one type of mindful eating – a technique that can be used to turn mealtimes into opportunities for meditation. Often when we're eating, we're not solely focused on the food itself, but on conversations or screens. However, it can help strengthen your mind–body connection to slow down – whether you're alone or with others – and bring all your awareness to your food.

For helping with sleep, this meditation is best practised in the evening.

TO PRACTISE MINDFUL EATING:

1. Sit down with your food without any distractions.
2. Take a few deep breaths, inhaling through your nose and exhaling through your mouth.
3. Continue to focus on your breathing as you look at your food with gratitude (consider, for example, how your vegetables grew in the sunshine or how the cookies you're eating were baked).

4. Slowly engage your other senses (What does your food smell like? How does your body feel in this moment?).

5. As you slowly try your food, gently close your eyes and observe the texture and flavour.

6. If your mind wanders, guide your thoughts back to nourishing yourself and hearing your body.

7. Once you're done eating, take a few more deep breaths while mentally scanning your body (see p.45) to see how you're feeling – by practising mindful eating, you'll be calmer and mentally prepared for good sleep.

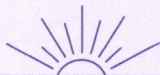

Variation: You can also incorporate mindfulness while you select or cook your food or snack.

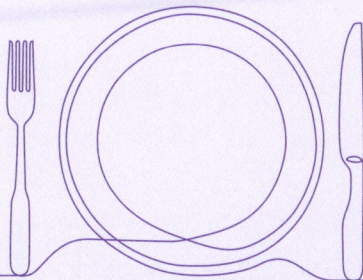

JOURNALLING
MEDITATION

LAW OF ATTRACTION

The law of attraction is a theory that our thoughts hold energy (positive or negative) that can correlate to our external experiences. To attract the things you want (like improved sleep), this journalling meditation is designed to help you reflect on and energetically match what you desire.

TO PRACTISE:

1. Find somewhere comfortable to sit where you will be able to write in a journal.

2. Sit or recline with your materials ready (a journal and something to write with).

3. Close your eyes, bringing your awareness to your breath for a few minutes.

4. When you feel ready, open your eyes and write down things you want for yourself (such as things related to sleep), and include how attracting these things (like restfulness, for example) would make you feel energetically.

5. Once you're done journalling, close your eyes again and tune into that desired energy, imagining what it would feel like to be relaxed, happy or refreshed, as if you've already unlocked your wants.

6. Continue visualizing yourself, including every sensory detail of where you want to be and how you hope to feel.

7. Inhale through your nose and exhale through your mouth.

8. Open your eyes.

VISION BOARD

Vision boards are mindfulness tools that can help you focus on your intentions throughout your day and while meditating. You can even create a vision board dedicated to improving sleep (and the process of creating one can be meditative in itself).

TO PRACTISE:

1. Find somewhere comfortable to sit where you will be able to write and create a collage.

2. Think of your intentions for this vision board and collect related images (to focus on sleep, consider using images of bedrooms from magazines, printing restful images or writing down quotes about dreaming).

3. With your images, words, quotes or any other visual elements ready, begin writing and collaging to create your vision board in a journal.

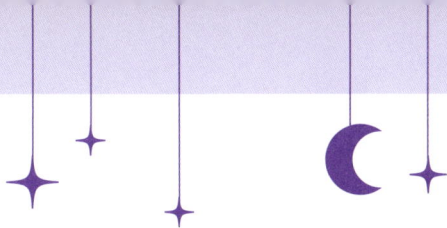

4. Let yourself be fully aware of how each image or word makes you feel as you collage; observe how your breath naturally slows as you focus on this meditative activity.

5. Once you're done creating your vision board, take the time to truly look at it and see what feelings the images or words you've chosen evoke.

6. Holding feelings of restfulness or sleepiness in your heart, close your eyes, bring your awareness to your breath and imagine how you would feel if this board was your reality.

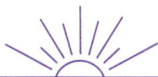

Variation: After finishing this meditation exercise, you can journal about anything you want to start doing to help your vision become reality. Feel free to create new vision boards whenever you'd like.

REFLECTING ON THE DAY

Writing in a tangible journal can help you reflect on your day in an intentional way and achieve a peaceful state of mind, serving as a meditation in itself or helping you wind down in the evening before a different meditation exercise. This particular journalling practice is for quietening busy minds or noisy thoughts around bedtime.

TO PRACTISE:

1. In the evening, find somewhere comfortable to sit where you will be able to write in a journal.

2. Sit or recline with your materials ready (a journal and something to write with).

3. On a blank page, write down a few reflective, guiding questions for yourself to answer – these can be questions you come up with yourself or things like: What made me happy

today? What caused me stress today? What would bring me joy tomorrow? Is there anything cluttering my mind? What energy would I like to bring into tomorrow?

4. Once you've written down a few questions for yourself, don't answer them immediately – instead, close your eyes and mentally reflect on them.

5. As you reflect, focus on your breath, inhaling through your nose and exhaling through your mouth.

6. After a few minutes, open your eyes and answer the questions with a quieter mind.

7. When you're done journalling, feel free to review what you wrote before closing your eyes again.

8. Bringing your awareness back to your breath, continue to meditate or allow yourself to drift off.

VISUALIZATION

LOVING-KINDNESS MEDITATION

Commonly encompassing two parts – receiving and sending – loving-kindness meditations are for enhancing interconnectedness. Feelings of kindness can tap into the parasympathetic nervous system (the "rest and digest" state in the body that is responsible for making you feel safe and calm) and help you to end your day on a compassionate note. As with any mindfulness practice, slowing down your heart rate and thoughts can help with sleep.

TO PRACTISE:

1. Get comfortable, gently close your eyes, and bring your awareness to your breath.

2. Begin visualizing receiving loving-kindness from someone who you feel loved or supported by, as if they're sitting before you and wishing you all the best.

3. After several minutes, breathe deeply and imagine sending loving-kindness to someone you know who could use extra love or support, as if they're sitting before you – inhale while thinking of your intention for them and imagine your wish reaching their heart as you exhale.

4. Continue focusing on these visualizations or integrate a mantra (see p.59) related to self-love or compassion for others.

5. Complete this meditation by bringing your awareness back to your physical sensations by taking three deep breaths then opening your eyes.

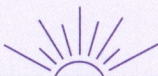

Variation: You can start by solely focusing on loving-kindness for yourself, and eventually integrate visualizing other people with practice.

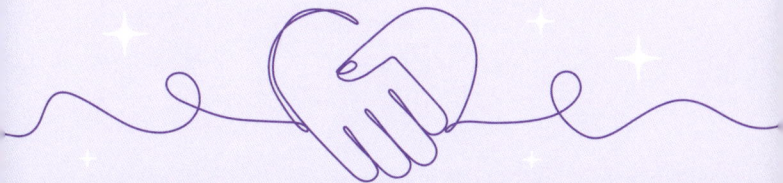

HEALTH AND
HEALING MEDITATION

The mind and body are intrinsically linked when it comes to our well-being. While sometimes our emotions can keep us from sleeping, at other times worries about our health or physical symptoms (like chronic pain) can be the preventative factor. Fortunately, mindfulness and meditation can be used to effectively manage both mental and physical stressors.

Often, imagery is used within healing meditations. Before practising this meditation, try to think of an image that could represent healing. You could visualize your immune system thriving like a luscious rainforest or maybe your physical symptoms transforming into something glorious – your visuals and imagery will be specific to you.

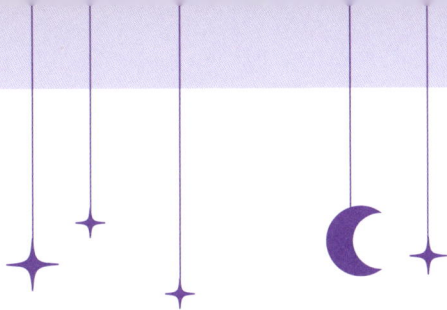

TO PRACTISE:

1. Inhale through your nose and exhale through your mouth, slowly closing your eyes as you relax.

2. With your eyes closed, scan your body to observe how you feel (see p.45).

3. Once you're tuned into your body, begin to focus on your chosen imagery, allowing the visualization to consume your thoughts.

4. As you visualize, imagine that the air you are inhaling is full of healing energy, and with every exhale you're cleansing your body of anything standing in the way of your well-being and sleep.

5. Complete this meditation with a mantra of your choice that affirms your intention to feel healed, enabling you to sleep.

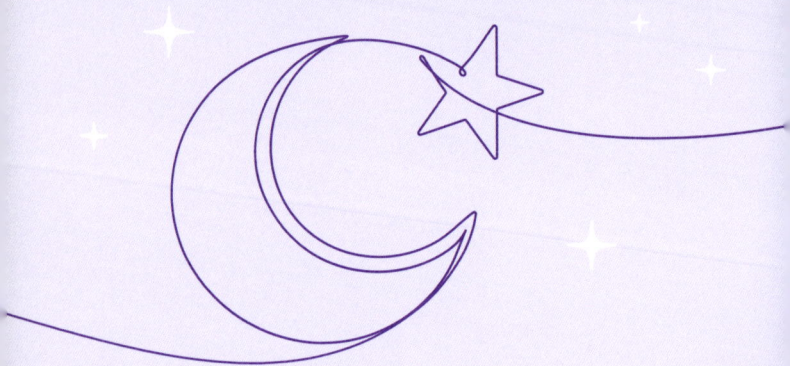

The best bridge between despair and hope is a good night's sleep.

E. JOSEPH COSSMAN

Sleep helps
you win at life.

AMY POEHLER

SOUND

You may have explored other sound-based meditations (see pp.56–7), but did you know there's a type of music designed to alter your brain frequency?

A binaural beat is music with two tones playing at different frequencies. Listening to binaural beats causes your brain frequency to change, matching that of the music. This helps you reach a desired mental state (useful for mindfulness and meditation).

Binaural beats can affect five different brain waves within different frequency ranges. While Delta waves are the lowest frequency state – associated with both sleep and meditation – you can learn about all of the ranges and some of their effects here:

- **Delta (1–4 Hz):** good for healing, meditation and sleep
- **Theta (4–8 Hz):** good for creativity, meditation and relaxation
- **Alpha (8–14 Hz):** good for focus, learning and positivity
- **Beta (14–30 Hz):** good for attention, cognition and energy
- **Gamma (30–100 Hz):** good for memory

TO PRACTISE:

1. Queue some binaural beats music online or on a music streaming platform.
2. Click play when you're ready to begin.
3. With the music playing, close your eyes and focus on your breathing – inhaling through your nose and exhaling through your mouth.
4. Let the music naturally guide the pace of your breathing.
5. Tune into the sounds, which can hopefully deepen your state of calm or lull you to sleep.

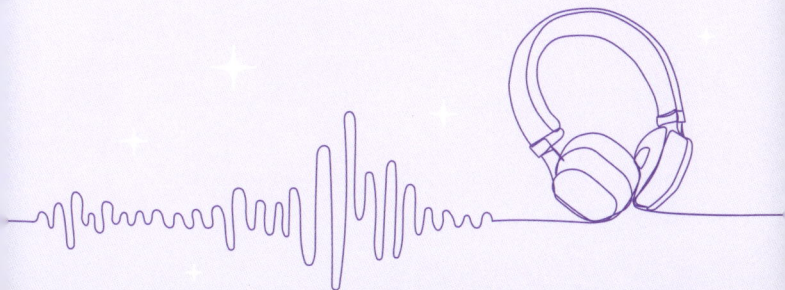

GRATITUDE MEDITATION

Gratitude meditation is a great practice to start your mornings or wind down at the end of the day. Shifting your focus toward gratitude should bring you a sense of calm which in turn can help improve your sleep.

TO PRACTISE:

1. In a comfortable position, close your eyes or keep them open with a soft focus on the space around you.

2. Take a few deep breaths, inhaling through your nose and exhaling through your mouth.

3. Allow your breath to return to normal and either think about the day ahead of you or reflect on the day behind you – observe what emotions come up. (Is it or was it a peaceful day? A stressful day? A happy day?)

4. Observe these emotions like clouds passing in the sky; let them float by without judgement or attachment.

5. As the clouds pass, bring your awareness to things you feel grateful for – try to think of as many as you can, beginning with the smallest things and then expanding outward toward people you're grateful for and the love in your life.

6. Allow this meditation to fill your heart with gratitude.

7. Know that the calm, happy feelings you gain by reflecting on the positives in your life will contribute to enhanced sleep.

CANDLE MEDITATION

Candle meditation (also known as "candle gazing meditation") or trataka *(yogic gazing) is an ancient Indian yogic practice. As the name suggests, this meditation technique involves gazing at a candle and can help improve focus, mental health and sleep quality.*

If you do not have a candle, you can use candle meditation videos online for this meditation.

TO PRACTISE:

1. Select your candle – any kind will work, but you can choose one that connects with your intention for this meditation (sandalwood, rose and lavender are commonly used scents and the colour of the candle can also have a particular meaning, see pp.68–9).

2. Sit or stand (with your back straight), placing your candle before you at eye level.

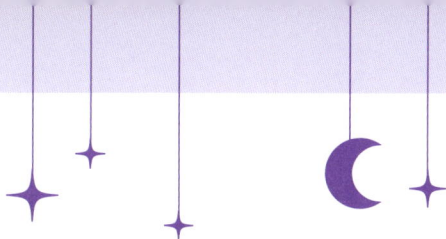

3. Begin by taking a few deep breaths – inhaling through your nose and exhaling through your mouth – while focusing on your intention.

4. Continue focusing on your breath as you light your candle.

5. Once it is flickering, follow the flame with your eyes – you may experience a strong connection with your third eye (a chakra or energy point in your body associated with intuition).

6. You can experiment with closing your eyes, focusing on inner light or the warm colours you may see through your eyelids – imagine that you're absorbing the light and love of the candle as you meditate.

7. When your meditation is finished, thank your candle, focusing on gratitude as you blow it out.

8. Take a few moments to rest, breathing with your eyes closed.

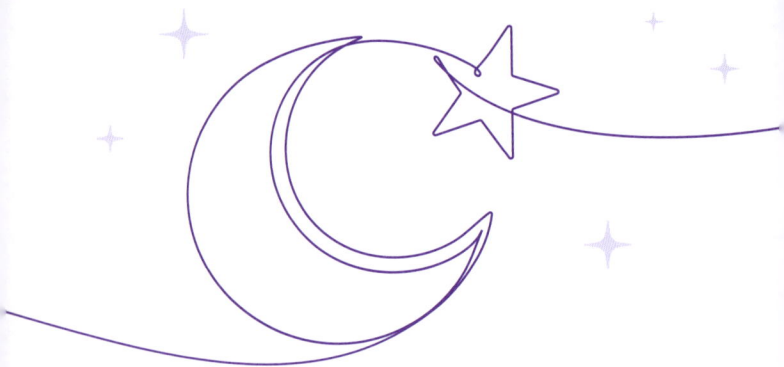

*Meditation showed
me how much
energy silence has.*

MADONNA

RECAPPING ON YOUR DAY MEDITATION

When we're caught up in our busy lives, we can experience racing thoughts at night that can make it hard to fall asleep. This meditation exercise helps you to review and reflect on your day so you can drift off more easily.

TO PRACTISE:

1. Sit or lie down before going to bed, close your eyes and focus on your breathing.

2. Slowly scan your body (see p.45).

3. Continue to breathe, becoming aware of your thoughts.

4. Gently guide yourself back to your morning, visualizing your breakfast and/or the clothes you put on.

5. Move on to your afternoon and then your evening – review everything you did during the day without judgement or lingering on one thing for too long.

6. Once you reach the present moment, fill your mind and heart with gratitude for yourself for taking the time and creating the space to meditate.

7. Allow your mind and body to rest as you fall asleep.

MANDALA MEDITATION

DRAWING YOUR OWN MANDALA

Beyond focusing on mandalas while meditating (see pp.74–6) or colouring them in to practise mindfulness (see pp.106–7), you can also experiment with drawing them yourself.

It's not important what these drawings look like. Whether you use simple shapes or explore intricate details, this activity will help you bring your awareness to your breath and mind–body connection.

TO PRACTISE:

1. Find a place where you will be comfortable to sit and draw.

2. Sit or recline with your drawing materials ready.

3. Close your eyes and set your intentions while inhaling through your nose and exhaling through your mouth.

4. When you're ready, open your eyes and allow your breath to follow the movement of your hand as you draw – you could start by drawing a circle, dividing it into four parts and colouring different designs in each quadrant. (Feel free to use the mandalas on pp.75–6 as a guide.)

5. Allow your thoughts to wander, observing the colours and shapes you're gravitating toward and how drawing changes your mental or emotional state.

6. Once you've finished, close your eyes again and end this meditation by inhaling gratitude and exhaling stress, knowing that this time you've dedicated to your practice will help to improve your sleep.

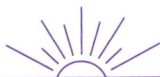

Variation: Combine drawing with breathwork (see pp.46–55), music (see pp.142–3), aromatherapy (see pp.60–1) and/or colour meditation (see pp.68–9).

MOVING MEDITATION

Studies have shown that physical activity and mindfulness are connected to improvements in sleep quality and overall well-being, and can therefore be helpful if you're struggling with insomnia or quietening your busy mind. Moving meditation involves slowly moving while meditating to bring your awareness to your body, your surroundings and your mind–body connection. The meditation can be practised indoors or outside at any time of day, while walking or in a chair.

TO PRACTISE:

1. Go somewhere you can move freely (your house, garden, neighbourhood, a park, a local trail, the beach, etc.).

2. Before incorporating movement, be completely still – feel the weight of your body, look at the space around you and take a few grounding breaths.

3. Return your breath to its natural flow and begin moving very slowly, pausing to take deep breaths.

4. Focus on the sensory experience – the sound of your movements, the smell and feeling of the air, or maybe the sights around you – maintaining awareness without lingering on any thoughts.

5. Notice how your body feels and what feelings or thoughts you're experiencing.

6. When your mind wanders, bring your awareness back to your movement and surroundings; the goal isn't to prevent thinking, but to observe your thoughts without judgement.

7. To complete this meditation, return to stillness and take a few deep breaths, knowing that this practice will aid better sleep.

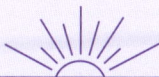

Variation: Moving meditation is often practised between sitting meditations, so feel free to begin or end this practice with other forms of meditation.

The thing about
meditation is,
you become more
and more you.

DAVID LYNCH

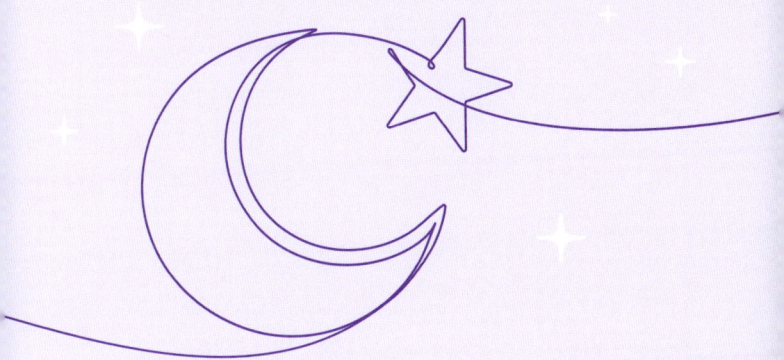

*Discover the great ideas
that lie inside us…
discover the power of sleep.*

ARIANNA HUFFINGTON

Farewell

Sleep is incredibly powerful and feeling well rested improves our overall well-being, allowing us to enjoy life more fully. When insomnia, physical symptoms, mental health or racing thoughts are keeping us up, it can be challenging to get back on track and feel rejuvenated. Fortunately, mindfulness and meditation have been shown to help with sleep, managing pain, reducing stress and fostering the mind–body connection.

Regardless of what may keep you from sleeping, hopefully you've discovered and explored new solutions in these pages. Practising the various tips and 5-, 10- and 15-minute mindfulness exercises and meditations throughout this book should help you to improve the quality of your sleep and

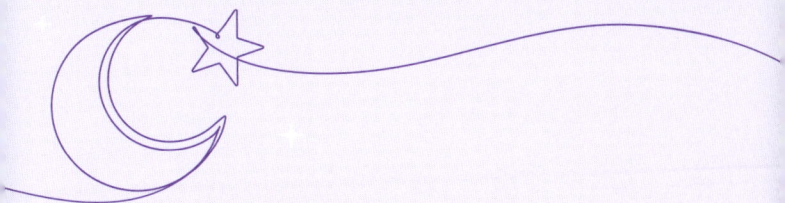

unlock the range of benefits meditation offers. Incorporating mindfulness and meditation into your daily life can of course lead to improvements beyond sleep and help you to feel more balanced, focused and peaceful overall.

Wishing you sweet dreams, self-love, compassion and joy on your journey to better sleep.

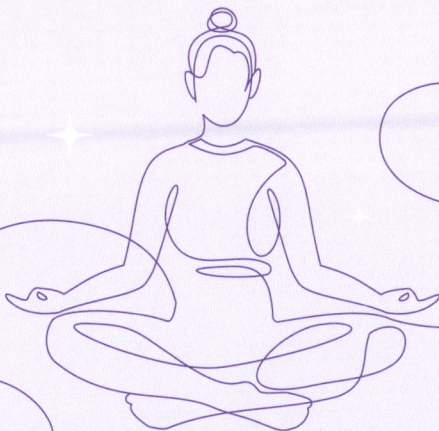

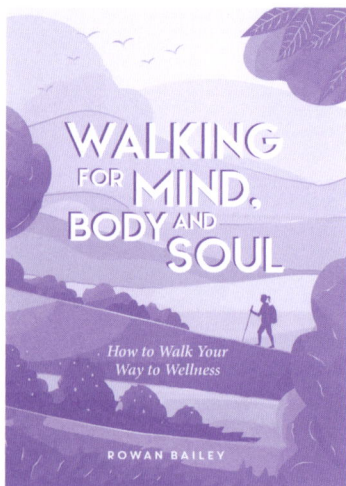

WALKING FOR MIND, BODY AND SOUL

HOW TO WALK YOUR WAY TO WELLNESS

Rowan Bailey | **Hardback** | **ISBN: 978-1-83799-516-5**

Guiding you through the physical, spiritual and sensory benefits of walking, these pages will help you reap the therapeutic wonders of putting one foot in front of the other. Bursting with practical tips, insightful information and inspirational ideas, this book is your companion to crafting a life of balance and bliss with every step.

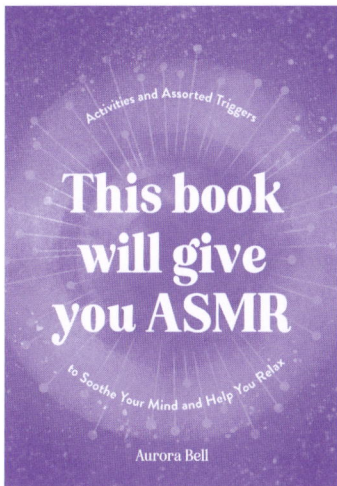

Activities and Assorted Triggers

This book will give you ASMR

to Soothe Your Mind and Help You Relax

Aurora Bell

THIS BOOK WILL GIVE YOU ASMR

ACTIVITIES AND ASSORTED TRIGGERS TO SOOTHE YOUR MIND AND HELP YOU RELAX

Aurora Bell | Paperback | ISBN: 978-1-83799-498-4

Tap into the tingly world of ASMR (Autonomous Sensory Meridian Response) and experience the soothing power of sound with this immersive activity book. Teeming with tips and exercises, this mesmerizing book will trigger your ASMR reactions. Whether you're tracing patterns or creating your own tingle-inducing tools, this book will give you ASMR.

Have you enjoyed this book?
If so, why not write a review on your favourite website?

If you're interested in finding out more about
our books, find us on Facebook at **Summersdale
Publishers**, on Twitter/X at **@Summersdale** and
on Instagram and TikTok at **@summersdalebooks**
and get in touch. We'd love to hear from you!

Thanks very much for buying this Summersdale book.

www.summersdale.com